WEIGHT

LOSS

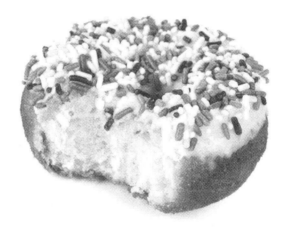

By
John
ASHWORTH

Copyright © 2012
John Ashworth

Published in the United States by

Insight Publishing

707 West Main Street, Suite 5
Sevierville, TN 37862
800-989-7771
www.insightpublishing.com

ISBN - 978-1-60013-913-0

10 9 8 7 6 5 4 3 2 1

This book is dedicated to my family, Laura, Carl, and Ana. Thank you for believing in me . . .

. . . and to my sister, Wendi, who backed down to no one.

Lastly, to Mrs. Bergman, who wanted to see my "name in print."

Nomad Victories

What you see here are entries over the last few years in what is known in my fitness studio as the *Nomad Victory Book*. I've included them in this book, because they represent the real-life example of the work I cover throughout this book. They represent real-life examples of small victories that accumulate over time and add up to success over the years.

So many people give up on weight loss because when the going gets tough, or they lose ground, and when they feel their results are not coming fast enough, they lose hope. We have been led to believe by popular culture and the media that weight loss should come quick and easy, and we allow ourselves this indulgence over and over again. The problem is that this belief is not realistic, and is not serving us very well at all.

In the context of your daily life and the challenges that lie therein, it is often extremely difficult to maintain the discipline it takes to lose weight and achieve success in your health and fitness. Especially inside a culture that doesn't necessarily support your efforts on a daily basis.

These victories represent the small changes that take place consistently over time when you stick with it. These small changes might not seem like much at the time, but when you add them, and write them down over the years, they represent BIG accomplishments, and that is what creates true and lasting personal transformation and weight loss.

I've left out the last names for privacy, but these are real people with real stories and real victories that they felt compelled to share along the way. I hope you enjoy them and are inspired by them as much as I am.

—John

P.S. I encourage you to create your own Victory Book and to document each success as it manifests, even if it seems a little silly at the time. Because I guarantee you that when you're struggling, taking time to look back on all the small things you've accomplished along the way is a valuable exercise in self-reflection that will help keep you going.

You can share your Nomad Victories if you like at
www.FitnessNomadVictories.com

The Fitness Nomad Victory Book Entries

"My stamina is so much better now. I pegged my heart rate at 160 beats per minute for 30 minutes last week. That wasn't possible when I first started."—*Jesse*

"I feel 10 times better! I have a ton more energy and I feel better about myself because now I know I'm doing something for myself."—*Sheri*

"I played 5 rounds of golf in 4 days, but my back did not bother me at all."—*Dale*

"I dropped 11 pounds and 10 blood pressure points in 3 months. I feel great!"—*Fritz*

"Since I've been working with John, my blood sugar level is back in the normal range, I've lost at least 12 pounds, and I've made a new friend."—*Sheri*

"Over the past 6 months or so, I've taken for granted how much stronger I've become. Today, as I was pounding it out on the elliptical machine, I had a flashback to when I first started with John over a year ago and how I was gasping and lightheaded after 7 minutes of cardio. Today I felt I could go for hours. The comparison made me Smile!" —*Laura*

"I'm getting a lot more physical since I started working with you. I used to work maybe an hour in my garden. Yesterday I was out for at least 2 hours without a problem. I was still getting tired but my attitude was totally different."—*Maggie*

"In just 3 weeks, the running, combined with the strength training I perform at the Fitness Nomad, has already made my legs a lot stronger. And my pants are fitting better already too!" —*Peggy*

"Since I've been exercising with John over the last year, I have not had nearly as many headaches as I used to get."—*Pat*

"I think I'm really kinda starting to get muscles!"—*Cherie*

"My decision to come here was a good one. I feel the best about myself that I've felt, since I had my stroke in "04."—*Mary*

"I'm the healthiest I've been in my life!"—*Deb age 49 (Not 50!)*

"I feel more fit than I've ever been. (since high school). I've also had a 5 to 6 percent drop in body fat in 2 months."—*Wade*

"One aspect I hadn't thought about was my posture. Since I've starting lifting, I'm walking & sitting straighter. I feel uplifted!" —*Cherie*

"My massage therapist says she can tell a definite difference in my muscle tone after working out for 3 months—and I now can do pushups!"—*Michelle*

"Since working out here, I feel more energized throughout my work day."—*Kathy*

"My legs are more shapely than they have ever been in my entire life!"—*Laurel*

"I've lost 9 pounds, 1 inch around my waist and 1 percent of my body fat in just one month. And I'm getting stronger and doing my cardio even when I don't want to. That is improvement!"—*Mark*

"After 2 days on my "pumped up" exercise program it looks like I have dipped down below my "stuck point" on the scale! I did a double take this AM."—*Love, Mom*

"I haven't worn a 38 waist pair of pants in 10 or more years! And that's what I'm going to buy tonight."—*Bill*

"I checked my blood pressure and it was 119/71. Best Ever!" —*Kathy*

"I hadn't been to Borders in about a year and I noticed that I wasn't out of breath at all climbing the stairs!"—*Tyler*

"I made it through the holidays with no weight gain; instead I lost 1.4% body fat!"—Char

"Okay, me again. This time I can report going from a size 12 to a size 8 slacks! Yahoo!!"—*Char*

"For the first time in a long time, I can reach all the way down and touch my toes."—*Cathy*

"Accomplishments: Have not eaten junk food within the last 5 weeks."—*Barb*

"Not an April Fool's gag: I lost 6 pounds in 6 weeks. My running has really paid off. Thank you, Mike & Scott!"—*Char*

"One year today of sweating, working hard, being supported, and finally, succeeding. This has been life-changing. Thank you Nomad staff & John!"—*Char*

"This is the longest I've stuck with an exercise program."—*Kelly*

"John said he's having the most fun in a long time. No, I am." —*Barb*

"I didn't expect that I was going to have fun when I signed up. Your staff is great and makes it fun!"—*Dennis*

"Before I started working out here I had significant lower back pain. After four weeks, all the pain is gone and I feel great. TNX."—*Dennis*

"My chiropractor said that "whatever you're doing keep it up.' It's much easier to adjust your back."—*Kristyn*

"I have not needed to see my chiropractor since starting here. When I began I thought I would have to see him more. I'm slowly adapting to this and enjoying it."—*Glenn*

"I just had the best 30 minutes of my life!"—*Kasia*

"I appreciate [enjoy might be too much :-)] your boot camp classes! I've grown stronger and more energetic since I started and that is my goal, so things are going well. When I end my stint in April or May, it is not a reflection on how it is going—it is just a reflection on what I can afford in the mix of kid obligations and the rest of my life." —*Best, Claudia*

"I feel 110 percent better! I'm more comfortable on my bike than I have been in a long time."—*Dani*

"Thank you so much for your teaching, your encouragement, and most of all for changing my approach to diet and exercise!"—*Dave*

"For the first time in a couple of years I can pick my son up and actually carry him up the stairs! It makes him very happy and me feel like the strongest Mom on Earth!"—*Dani*

"I have been at this now for five weeks. Today I tried a pair of pants that I was not able to wear because of some belly fat that was put on over the winter. Today I took those pants off the hanger and was able to fasten them with no problem. Thanks guys! Bring it on!"—*Jerry*

"A year ago, when I started at Fitness Nomad it took 2 guys to put our sailboat away. Both guys would lift the boat toward the rafters to be hung. This year I was able to lift the boat myself!"—*Greg*

"This is good. I'm doing weights. I feel real!"—*Liz*

"Thanks to 6 months of boot camp Fall Hunting in Montana was a breeze!"—*Ally*

"My energy level has already doubled. I'm sleeping better and I'm more cheerful."—Suzanne

"Thank you for the difference you've each made in my life."—*Amy*

"I haven't been sick all year!"—*Michael*

"Thanks for your support and positive attitude. I truly enjoy coming in to work-out!"—Maureen

"I've really enjoyed and I've accomplished a lot of my goals. I lost 25 pounds! Thanks so much for boot camp!"—*Ally*

"I'm new and I LOVED class (Boot Camp) yesterday, feel very energized (and only moderately achy) today, and will definitely be back."—*Judy*

"I used to have headaches 3 to 4 days per week and now I only get about 1 a month!"—*Maureen*

"I placed 31st in my age group and 316th out of 12,800 runners. I cut a minute off my personal record. The Nomad helped me get there."—*Dan*

"I always feel better when I come here . . ."—*Tom*

"I feel so much more energized now that I've started. I can't remember the last time I just got right out of bed without trouble. Yes! It's been challenging to fit it in but it's worth it!"—*Jenny*

INTRODUCTION

Weight Loss—

The Job No One is Training You For

I just finished listening to an interview with Michael Moore, filmmaker and author of the best-selling book, "Here Comes Trouble" on NPR's Talk of the Nation.

My wife, Laura, says that he reminds her of me. That makes me feel really good. I'm eternally grateful for Laura's belief in me over the years. Laura didn't have to say why. I know why. I've *never* been afraid to tell it like it is. Well, that's not fair, of course I've been afraid—lots of times—and in many cases shaking with emotion that you can literally hear in my voice, but I *never* let that stop me.

Unfortunately, this trait—a trait I call "undying passion"—often leaves me groping for friends, like a blind man who has lost his seeing-eye dog. I don't like to hold back, and I can't stand it when others do the same or aren't being up-front with me. I can always tell. It literally makes me feel ill, and during times in my life when I've been holding back far too much than someone should have to, it often leads to depression. So if I have to make a choice between friends and avoiding depression and stomach aches, I'll choose passion any day. And if I'm being completely honest with you (which I always am), I'll also tell you that I don't worry too much about your reaction.

Once again, this trait, and these beliefs and convictions in my life have not always served me swimmingly in my career as a fitness professional. The problem for me is that if you say something that I think is nonsense, I'm going to call you out on it—just as I would expect you to do the same for me. Unfortunately, most people would rather sit on their instincts, and let them incubate, forever maybe, as long as they don't have to be uncomfortable. For a life that is so darn short, fleeting, and precious in its rarity, I often wonder why we make so much time for indecision, denial, and passive aggressiveness.

Accountability

I've started this book with the statements above and with a brief discussion about Accountability for one very important reason. This kind of honesty and openness to being human, and accepting yourself and those you come in to contact with in life, is at the heart of your overall success as a human being, no matter how you define that success. This includes your success in your effort to improve your health and fitness, lose weight, and transform your body; if that is, in fact, what you desire.

I've qualified that last statement for an important reason—a reason explained by an important insight I've experienced first-hand as a fitness coach during the last two decades. There is one simple ingredient common to those individuals who achieve weight loss and body transformation success, and it has *nothing* to do with whether or not they had breakfast this morning. The clients who have the most success are the ones who remain open to the process, and at the core of their pursuit of what I like to call peak health is a drive to improve as a human being—a drive to keep going no matter how big an obstacle they run into along the way. Believe me when I tell you that *big* obstacles and sticking points are *always* part of this process. Remember, it will be your response to these obstacles that shapes your outcome.

You hear a lot of talk in our everyday media, and in our culture, about all the problems that create the perfect storm for obesity—too much easy access to unhealthy food, sedentary jobs and lives, stress, unsupportive spouses, colleagues, friends, or family members. Sure, none of these surface level obstacles make it any easier, but at the core of this process, and your ability to grow as a human being, is your sheer willingness to make it happen, in spite of any circumstance, problem, or seemingly insurmountable obstacle.

Think about it for a moment . . . though only a minority in our culture are physically active (only 5 percent), those fitness enthusiasts who find a way to do this, do it in spite of everything that stands in their way. They *choose* to rise above their circumstances, drive right past the Taco Bell on the way home, and prepare a beautiful, healthy, nutritious, home-cooked meal even though it will also mean that they are up until 9:30 or 10 doing the dishes that come with it. This is a *choice* they make, night after night. What choices are you making?

The first step in this process is a willingness to be held accountable for your action or inaction, whatever the case might be—willingness to check-in, and get *present* with your current state of affairs. There, is an even stronger will to accept your failures as they arrive, make the necessary adjustments, and then keep going. Remember, your success in any aspect of your life boils down not to luck or circumstance, but instead to your own personal *reaction* to your world around *you*.

Inside this book I will share stories of clients who ran away when the going got tough. I will talk about belief systems and why they are so important, and I will share a number of short stories with you that center around what it truly takes to lose weight and transform your body. Keep in mind, too, that regardless of your weight loss and body transformation goals, there are many other positive and important benefits that come from embarking on this journey that we like to call health and fitness. So, even if your weight loss goal is small, or you don't want to focus on that particular aspect of the work, it's okay—there is still a lot for you here. After all, very often it is a client's unbalanced pursuit of outcome change that often derails his or her progress before anything else.

In other words, it is easy to become transfixed on a perceived need to see the dial move, when in fact, in order to get that dial to move, you are likely to find many other challenges more pressing for attention. These are details that will be important for your overall and long-term success in this effort—a job that, as I indicated in the title of this book, No one is training you for.

Be realistic

"Please, I beg you, don't let this happen to you—be realistic . . ."

—John

The story I'm about to share with you here is important. It's important because it shows us a belief system that is feeding the unfortunate "virus" our culture has contracted. Every time this happens, it makes me just a little sicker to my stomach.

I met with a client about a week ago to do a regular review of the numbers—the usual stuff: body fat percent, weight, waist, and hip circumference. This person had been working with me for about five months. Unfortunately that work came to an abrupt end on an idle Tuesday morning. It was the direct result of a problem that plagues a culture obsessed with immediate gratification and the mismatch between the current level of action, effort, and adherence, and expectations about how far the dial should be moving.

These interactions are always frustrating for me. As time passes, however, I am allowed a view with much more objectivity. It has now become an excellent opportunity to touch on something very important to your weight loss and body transformation efforts—your belief system.

The client was suddenly devastated by the fact that *none* of the outcomes had moved very much at all over the five-month training and coaching period. Despite the fact that that this client reported "I can now wear a pair or two of pants I haven't fit into in awhile." The fact that the "Official Dial" on the scale and body fat machine did not move more, was ultimately enough to send this person reeling like a spoiled little kid who doesn't want to come home for dinner.

As the coach, the lack of movement on the dial did not bother or surprise me one bit. It was obvious to me that this client wasn't being completely forthright in her reporting. This is something that research demonstrates is a constant problem—an underreporting of how much one eats, and over-reporting of how much one exercises. It seems like human nature to me.

In fact, this person's logs were nonexistent. That fact, coupled with perfect verbal reports, *always* mean one thing. Sure, the client knows what she is supposed to be doing, but the client is not doing it and she doesn't want to tell me. Still fine with me on most levels because I know there is always a chance that the client will eventually come around. This is part of the game of coaching—it's a dance. Not a waltz, though. It's much less graceful at times.

Regardless, the client had been working hard, and had accomplished things far more important at this point than getting the dial to move. Things like establishing a regular exercise program in spite of a tremendously hectic work and travel schedule, improved levels of strength and conditioning, better back control, a more positive and grounded mental outlook (as noted by the client *and* her therapist), improved levels of self-confidence, better sleep, better nutrition at home and on the road, and so forth. Forget about the numbers, this client is on the way to living better and being healthier.

Believe me, we were a long way from being finished with all the work at hand, but we were making excellent progress and this person let a small thing like the scale completely destroy that progress. Please, I beg you, don't let this happen to you—be realistic.

The other thing people almost *never* do (at least immediately) in this situation, is consider it a victory that the dial did *not* move further in the wrong direction. Imagine what might have happened to this person's numbers during the last five months if the client had continued eating candy all day long at work, continued to not exercise, continued skipping so many meals during the day that the client was forced to wake in the middle of the night to eat, and so on. Likely the small up-titration of the numbers might not have even been noticed (mainly because of the lack of connection with the body), but that's exactly how it sneaks up on all of us over the years. One bad habit at a time, compounded over time, until one day we wake up with reflux in the middle of the night and finally decide to do something about it.

The problem is that in cases like this one, the disconnection between mind and body is so *vast*, that the client truly expects everything to reverse and change in an instant, or in this case five months. And if that doesn't happen, clients like this one very often run away from their coach. If it takes you twenty years to pack on thirty pounds and you can get those pounds off in just two to five years, I would say that is pretty darn good. But very often, that's not what we want to hear and definitely not what we are willing to accept as success in the moment. And the part that makes it even more insane is that not only do many people expect it to happen faster than that, they expect transformative results in minimum time with minimal effort. That's simply a recipe for insanity.

And when those quick results don't come, and the reality of the work at hand finally starts to settle in to the psyche, whom do you think many of these clients want to blame? That's right, yours truly.

Often, I can coach you down off that ledge after you calm down. I can help you connect with all of the positive benefits you have experienced, along with the fact that if you really are in this for the long run (the rest of your life), what you have accomplished thus far really is tremendous and, in this case, a fitting beginning to a long journey.

Unfortunately, I'm not always successful and the client quits. In an instant of insanity that makes for an interesting story, five months of hard work to build a foundation from which to build on is wasted.

At any rate, I got on this topic both because it helps me to write about it and because I read something else my wife, Laura, shared with me that helps illustrate my point even more clearly. The fact that just because you lower your cholesterol by 30 percent, doesn't mean you reduce your risk by 100 percent—there is still work to do. Heck, there is always work to do. The key is in your willingness to keep doing the work and to keep showing up and being present. That's where success really comes. Your faith in the process, in yourself, and in your coach is essential. And what's most essential is that in those moments where you get scared, frustrated, confused, bored, or whatever other obstacle might present itself to you, keep going. You keep working it until you find the solution. That's how big problems are solved, and that's how people achieve success.

If you hit a few obstacles, then just decide to turn around; you'll certainly get home safely, but all of your problems will still be there to greet you at the door.

The other night my daughter, Ana, asked me...

"Is there such a thing as perfect?"

Then a few nights ago she lifted her shirt at the dinner table and asked me a different question, "Am I fat?"

Ana is eight—a second grader.

Recently, it seems to be the topic of choice at the dinner table—fatness. And finally, the other night I asked that we put a stop to it. "Too much talk about fatness," I said. "Isn't there something more interesting we can discuss?"

Of course, part of it could be my fault. I'm a fitness guy, and very often spend time around the dinner table prophesying about what we need to do to solve the problem I see firsthand everywhere I look. In fact, one image that stands out in my mind are the dads I see at Ana's soccer games. Dutifully moving around the soccer field in an attempt to keep the second-graders on the ball during the game, I'm disturbed by how much belly fat I see hanging around under T-shirts and no longer hidden so well underneath dress clothes.

While it's true, we are all getting too fat, there is another problem brewing under the surface like a geyser. And once in awhile, that geyser gushes forth and douses us in a hot and sobering bath. All this focus on fatness, it turns out, can also make us quite self-conscious, confused, and ultimately sick with skinniness.

Here in Madison, NBC 15 news anchor Leigh Mills produced a story in 2011 that showed us firsthand how the problem of obesity can move 180 degrees in the opposite direction. In short, her story was that of a young girl who almost killed herself with an overemphasis on being skinny.

Please don't mistake my intent here. "Overweightness" is not off the hook. If you're too heavy, you certainly should be doing something about it because if you're not, well, your consequences are coming.

What I'm here to discuss instead is the vital importance of finding balance in our pursuit of health, fitness, weight loss, and a body image we can sleep with at night.

In my humble and professional opinion, I think we miss an important opportunity *every* day to educate our children about the importance of a good, wholesome, well-rounded pursuit of a more healthful lifestyle. We feed them garbage in the school lunch program, take away recess when we want to punish them, play movies, and eat sweets in the gymnasium when it rains, and discourage running on the blacktop because it's "unsafe."

In addition, we hold bake sales, and birthday parties, and feed them high glycemic food after soccer games, filling their everyday life with the idea that treats and sweets and other unhealthy food choices are acceptable and part of what it means to be a kid. And then we turn around and tell them fat is no good? Well, that's just confusing, even to me.

When a young girl is eating no more than a few bites of a cucumber and exercising for hours each day, and no one notices until she's on her death bed (from the story reported by Leigh Mills), you might be quick to say that she is an anomaly—a rare occurrence of imbalance that exists in stark contrast to what is *normal*. I'm not really here today to debate that with you. What I'm here to do today instead is to challenge you, as always.

I want to challenge you to reconsider your opportunity—*our* opportunity. The opportunity we miss *every* day when we don't sit down with our children for dinner to enjoy a meal that takes us longer than fifteen minutes to prepare, and probably three times as long to clean up. We have an opportunity every day in the school lunch room, not just to serve better food, but to also use that time to educate kids about good health, beyond their weight. How much do you think you could teach a group of kids if you spent ten minutes every day at lunch serving them stuff that could actually be considered food, and then teaching them what's in it, why it's so good for them, and how to sit down with intention and eat it? Ten minutes a day for twelve or thirteen years adds up to a lot; but we miss it, ignore it, and deny its importance.

Where's the balance?

In a world where we create shows like the *Biggest Loser,* we are also creating the exact opposite extreme in young girls like the one mentioned above.

The balance is in education. I see it every day with the clients I work with at my fitness studio. They don't know how to eat, exercise, and take good care of themselves. Many of them don't even know how to cook. Yes, we all are aware on some level that we need to work toward better health. And some of us even have some basic knowledge about how to do that. But ask someone you know if he or she actually put a meal plan together this week, or if the person knows what's for dinner tonight, and you will get a look with an expression I've seen a thousand times.

People will tell you they're too busy, tired, or confused to do the right thing. Some of them will tell you they don't even care. And if they won't tell you that, they're simply in denial. All of this is easy to ignore until we discover our daughter, lying in her hospital bed, fighting for her life, and for no good reason other than the fact that she thought she needed to be skinnier, perfect, or mostly, *not fat.*

The time has come for all of us to take responsibility for what we have all created together. The time has come for us to stop making excuses and to stop pretending that we don't have to do better. Because *every* day that goes by in our homes, in our schools, at our soccer games, and in the deep and personal crevices of our emotional lives that we don't take the opportunity to live better, be healthier, and find a reasonable balance in our pursuit of health is a day we miss to make a difference, not just for our children, but for all of us—for humankind.

I think we can all agree that we have some big problems to solve here. But what are we really doing about it?

What's for dinner tonight?

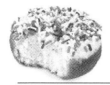

CHAPTER ONE

BELIEF SYSTEMS

What Do You Believe?

It might be more productive to ask you why you believe it, or how you came to believe what you believe today. What information or experience did you draw from to now draw the conclusions you are presenting me with today? Very often, those beliefs are not only inaccurate, but they are false, based on misinformation, and they are not serving you very well.

I want to start this chapter by sharing a recent and personal experience that has left me more sure than ever that your belief systems are vital to success in anything.

For my son, Carl's, first year of club soccer, I agreed to take on the responsibility of coaching his team. It was a paid position that would take me away from the fitness studio a couple of days per week, but that fits with my overall mission as a fitness professional and a dad. As it happens occasionally with clients too tied to old, worn out, and inaccurate belief systems, this experience did not turn out well, for me or for Carl.

Young athletes at this stage in their development need a special kind of care and coaching to begin teaching them the responsibility necessary to play club level soccer. When I say "responsibility" I don't just mean showing up for practice on time (although this was in fact one of the great challenges). What I meant was the responsibility of accepting the fact that this is no longer recreational. This is serious, competitive play where the emphasis is not on winning, but on being accountable to develop as boys, soccer players, and human beings. The experience is designed to provide them the opportunity to become skilled enough and disciplined enough to move on to higher levels of play as soccer players, if they are good enough.

The sad part of this situation was that the parents had other, more personal, self-centered, and destructive beliefs about what this experience should hold. In the end, they ruined it for me and for their children. Worse, they not only missed an opportunity for their kids to grow as people, but they missed an opportunity to instill a more positive, healthy, and well-balanced belief system in their children when it comes to competitive sports, and more importantly, the challenges of life.

The parents wanted to win, and at all costs. They wanted to believe that if we would just listen to them, and "tell their kids EXACTLY what to do" that they would at least be able to score a goal or two and prevent a "shutout." If we would just make sure they knew EXACTLY what they needed to do, when they needed to do it, and for how long, somehow this would make up for their inherent lack of skill, focus, and fitness.

The problem was that the parents' beliefs about what was happening and what needed to be done about it were completely erroneous. They made ignorant pleas that existed in stark contrast to youth soccer guidelines at this age level, mostly because they lacked any accurate knowledge about the game of soccer and how to develop ten-year-old players into club-level soccer competitors. In addition, it was their belief that we should "rescue" these kids from what turned out to be a very challenging, competitive environment.

The parents, at least for now, believe that rescuing their kids from a tough situation is a better way to solve the problem, versus using an incredibly difficult challenge as an opportunity to grow, mature, and be more ready for what comes next in their young lives. Not too dissimilar from a client's willingness to push just a little harder during each set of a strength training workout. Or, to work just a little harder to make sure and plan nutritious meals for their family each week.

The same thing happens to clients in the early stages of their training and coaching programs.

They believe they should be losing weight a lot faster, even though they are not adhering to the program 100 percent. They believe they should be able to lift more weight, even though they have no basis for comparison. They believe I should change their appointments at the last minute because holding them accountable to their personal schedule is just too difficult. They believe that results should come easy, simply because they decided to sign up and invest some time and money.

To you, the reader, I'm sure it is obvious that these beliefs do not serve any of these individuals well in their lives. And yet it's likely, in fact almost certain, that you have done the same thing when it comes to your weight loss and to other challenging situations in your life. No, you likely didn't impede the work of a professional the way the parents did in the story above, but yes, you held on to some belief, thought process, anger, frustration, resentment, or anxiety that prevented you from achieving what you said you wanted to achieve.

When clients get frustrated in their work with me, I always head straight for the accountability system. This is a piece of software I've developed that allows me an objective means of checking in on adherence to that which I know is essential for weight loss results. What is the first thing you think I find there when I go looking? You guessed it, not much, or not enough.

You can adhere closely to your nutrition program for five days per week, but for the two days you didn't, you often undo the benefits from those first five days. But what if you believe this shouldn't matter? Well, then I really can't help you, which brings me to probably the most important part in this section of the book. If I'm going to be able to help you, you have to believe that I can. And even when things get tough, that belief has to remain intact. Because what if it doesn't? If it doesn't, then we get nowhere, you get frustrated, and often you go looking for scapegoats (if not a different coach). Scapegoats can come in many forms including your current coach, your work schedule, your spouse, your children, your dog, your home inspection running late, your inability to say no, your unwillingness to get up earlier or stay up a little later, etc. The list is endless. It always will be. The only question is whether or not you believe you can rise above it.

Beginner's Mind

Every assignment, grand or tiny, should enlighten you. All you have is this moment. And if this moment is frightening, boring, unmanageable, unwanted, uncomfortable, excruciating, painful, or bland, well, then *renew!*

There is a concept that my yoga teacher has shared with me on more than one occasion and that I have learned elsewhere as well. It is known as "Beginner's Mind." Learning to approach every moment in this way is a great form of renewal. Otherwise, you will likely find yourself often stuck in old patterns of reaction that are merely a product of old worn-out belief systems. Destroying and forgetting what you did before is what allows you to carry on and create new things. Begin a new life, a new project, a new business venture, or a new job. Maybe even a new relationship with a loved one. For me recently, it was with my new dog, Allie—a great new walking partner.

This is the essence of life.

During winter time, especially here in Wisconsin in February, it is often difficult to find that sense of renewal amid the dead and frozen landscape. And this makes it tough to see new life, even though it is there, only waiting for the sun to burn a little warmer so that it can rise. Think about that for a second. All those seeds, just waiting for the right amount of sunlight. That's it. That's all they need to come alive.

What do you need to do to come alive?

The same holds true for your spirit. Life and contentment reside within you *all* the time. I know, it's hard to believe, which is one of the reasons for all my yoga practice. No matter how bad I might be feeling, no matter how disjointed, "gunky," worn out, and tired I might feel, Yoga brings me back to the moment, helps me release unwanted tension, and then I can begin again—I renew! This is where the true challenge sits, waiting for your arrival, right here in your ability to heat it up when it goes cold and lies dormant, often keeping you awake at night. What is it that you need to do about it? What is it in this moment that you will do to *renew!*

Tackling even a novel task that is new to you creates new synapses. This is one of the reasons regular exercise is so good for you. Your body is forced to renew during every workout, especially during your recovery. And every one of those workouts brings fresh blood, oxygen, and nutrients to cells that were dormant until you moved them. Every one of your new movements, thoughts, and actions, creates out of nowhere an electrical impulse that moves you.

Where will you allow these impulses to lead you?

Belief Systems—A Personal Example

I heard someone say the other day to my nine-year-old son, "It's a Man's World, Carl. That's just the way it is . . ."

Hogwash!

That might be what you believe, and that's fine, but it's not okay to make attempts to pass it along, especially to my nine-year-old son. That's irresponsible, and a great example of how a belief system can hold you back.

Often, my weeks take on a theme. It almost always happens. This week that theme has to do with Belief Systems—the set of beliefs anyone holds around any topic. Your belief systems guide you—good or bad.

What do you believe? And maybe more importantly, how are your belief systems working for you?

For any area of your life where you're struggling, document the belief systems that got you there, keep you there, and prevent you from moving forward. Because I'll guarantee you, that if you're stuck, your belief systems need attention. They almost always do because in order to grow, learn, create success, and truly live, you *must* refine your belief systems.

Here's a very personal example:

When I started this book, it wasn't exactly clear to me when it would land on your nightstand, and that was a good thing because then I worried less about how this story might affect a current client's image of my business. Toward the end of my tour in the Middleton studio, business was not going well at all. It hadn't really gone that well for about three years. The problem started when the economy took a dive in 2008. If you took a close look at the numbers, what you would see is a slight but steady drop in the number of new clients acquired on average each month and each quarter until the time I sold that studio.

"I feel like I'm reliving the life of my parents," Laura, my wife, had said to me during that time, "always struggling financially . . ." I agreed with her and decided not to go into any detail at the time. She was right, and I knew I wanted to do something about it, but didn't have a solution at that time.

I learned nothing about money, finances, and how to be a good businessman from my family and my father, who owned his own printing business for a time. He ran that business on old equipment, with no real bookkeeping, and no real clear vision as far as I could tell. The one thing I remember clearly was how often we seemed to be checking the mail to see if "The big check" was there so we could pay the bills and buy some groceries. There are plenty of other money stories like the following: we're driving around in a car that literally has threads showing on the tires because my Dad either hasn't taken care of it out of complete disregard, or doesn't quite have the money in the budget this week. Probably more the latter, but it didn't leave me very confident when it came to the concept of abundance.

These kinds of experiences have a way of forming belief systems about money, business, and family life. Even though I think consciously about these experiences while navigating my own life, somehow, I can see hints of similarities all around me. I don't like what I see, and I've decided to do something about it. Can you guess what is at the core of this process?

That's right—my belief systems.

Imagine the difficulty in committing to self-publish my book, and invest in two thousand copies up front at a time when it was extremely unclear as to whether or not we would survive the economic mess that had been created, both by our economy and by my own mistakes, indecisions, and poorly managed finances in the early stages of this business. Also imagine, that if I believed that sharing this with you would hurt my business and my brand, I'd just keep it to myself and you wouldn't have the benefit of learning from it.

I've invested almost half a month's bottom line in a project that has the potential to earn a lot more for me. Not just if I sell all two thousand copies of the first book, but also in the opportunity that is likely to follow now that it is done. I've dumped half my monthly bottom line into a project that I'm still trying to find enough time for, but which I believe is vital to our survival as a family business. It's vital, however, only if I believe in what this project and its exposure can do for me and my fitness career. Because it would be just as easy not to believe in it and worry incessantly if I should publish it all.

Every day, I have to work on strengthening my belief system around this project and its potential to help me grow my business, evolve personally, and advance my career. Because every day, there are voices in my head that would love to sabotage the effort. "What if you don't sell any of the books, John?" "What if everyone says your writing sucks and you should give it up?" "What if *nothing* good comes of it?" What if— What if— What if— You get the idea, and I'll bet you can completely relate to *exactly* what I'm talking about, because we all do it. We all have that part of our brain. It's what Seth Godin calls the "Lizard Brain" (See www.43folders.com /2010/01/26/godin-linchpin).

But your "Lizard Brain" can only do this to you if you allow it to happen . . .

It will be interesting to see what happens now that this book is finally finished. More importantly, it will be interesting to see how I react to its success or lack thereof. The non-lizard part of my brain tells me that it is this project—this first book—that will catapult me into the second half of my career and open doors and create opportunities that I couldn't even see before. But in order for this to happen, I *must* believe . . .

A big part of what makes this such a challenge is the part about "What if people say your writing sucks?" Since writing is what I love to do most, and is the thing I want to spend the second half of my career doing a lot more of, that particular fear is the one that creeps in the most. Because when I do finish this book, and send it out into the world, it might just *flop,* and then to keep going will be an even more difficult barrier to break through. But in order to get to that point, I've got to finish this book, and put it out into the world. And in order to finish this book, I *must* believe in this book. And then, regardless of what happens, I benefit from the fact that I held to my belief system, finished the book, and kept moving forward—something I see so many of my unsuccessful clients unable and unwilling to do.

Your Destiny and Your Evolution—

they are both up to you . . .

I like being in control of my own destiny. It's like having constant accountability for your personal growth. Because when you get right down to the bottom of your barrel, the truth is that your income can only grow to the extent that you do. And all of us have our old and often cumbersome belief systems to contend with in this deep dark place. I know I do, as I've shared with you earlier.

Personally, and until I found my writing groove, and decided to believe in its potential, I used to forge a battle from time to time between wanting to be an entrepreneur and wanting to let "The MAN" take care of me. If you're a business-owner like me, I'm sure you too have experienced those times during your work where you consider the possibility of what it might be like once again to let someone else worry about all the stuff you're working on today. This is normal. This is also, of course, opportunity for more growth.

You can't be brave if you're not scared; and you can't grow if everything is handed to you day after day, or if you're *never* presented with obstacles that challenge you. Once again, that's what exercise is all about—asking your body to get better by challenging it to do more. Sure, you can live in mediocrity for as long as you desire. I guarantee you that no one will notice, and that you'll have plenty of company there. Hiding in your cubicle where no one can see you is easy to do. But eventually the walls of that fake little office will begin to stink of the Chinese glue that holds them together. Or maybe they won't, and what you will find instead is the rest of your life rotting away in neglect.

I realize that not all of you are entrepreneurs. Some who read this will think, "Geez, I like my job, and I enjoy and am passionate about the work I do." To you I say, congratulations, you have found your place in the world and if you are truly content, then I am jealous. Because at the root of a good life is contentment. And if you're grounded enough, you can find that almost anywhere when you are being true to yourself.

The challenge for an entrepreneur like me is that contentment is not grounded in a day job. Contentment for me is the challenge I face every day of staying present with my destiny, my ideas, my undying pursuit of constant evolution as a human being, and my belief systems—the belief systems I've decided to keep. I know, that might sound like a bit much, but it *is* how I feel, which is why when a client asks me if he or she can skip their last set, leave class ten minutes early, have a cheat day, or any other self-limiting behavior, my answer is always the same:

"The degree to which you desire to thwart your evolution as a human being is entirely up to you."

Once again, what is it that *you* believe *you* need to do to evolve today?

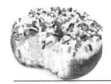

Chapter Two

The Problem

Most People Are Not Eating Enough!

Most people I work with as a fitness professional are gaining weight because they're eating too little, not too much. That's right! You read that correctly. If you're struggling to get lean, *you* are likely *not eating enough!* Allow me to explain.

First, let's not start any rumors, okay? The only way people can gain weight is by taking in more calories than their body needs on a consistent basis. That's the *only* way!

Well, okay, there is one other way to get fatter, but it doesn't show up on the scale. Cut your calories back far enough and your body will begin breaking down muscle to get what it needs. Your scale weight might not change much, but your body fat will be increasing as a result. Had your body fat checked lately?

Weight loss or weight gain is an energy balance equation: Energy in, energy out. Weight is gained when you take in more calories than your body needs to do the work it does every day (including your exercise). Those extra calories have no use, and hence, your body converts them to fat. It's the equivalent of taking the stuff that won't fit into your garage anymore to a storage space. Or, the equivalent of all that extra space that used to exist down in your basement, but has since been filled with all kinds of excess junk you don't even recognize anymore.

Think about that last example for a moment, though, and you'll begin to understand what I mean by the statement that you're not eating enough. If your basement or your storage space is now full of excess junk, it is likely that you don't pack excess stuff away there anymore. You're out of room. Instead, you get motivated on a Saturday morning, and get to work cleaning your basement, but by noon you realize that the job is much *bigger* than you thought, so you promise to get back to it later.

Life gets busy and you don't get back to it for another six months, at which time you realize that during that time period, you have refilled that space again with more excess junk. Somehow, the fullness of your basement or your storage space stays pretty even over time, in spite of your efforts to clean it out once in awhile.

Your efforts to lose weight are much the same as this process of cleaning the basement. Surprisingly, *most* clients I work with are literally *not* eating enough day by day to sustain their current metabolic rates and activity levels. They skip breakfast, miss meals like snacks, eat other unbalanced meals here and there throughout the day, and by dinner time, have severely undercut the number of calories they need to that point in the day.

Now, of course, if you're overweight, you find a way to make up those extra calories somewhere. Usually, it's in the form of empty calories like alcohol, sugar, simple carbohydrates, and larger meals consumed late in the day at dinner and afterward, as your body makes an attempt to make up for the lack of nourishment throughout the day. Many busy business professionals in particular, skip a lot of meals during the week while ignoring the body's need for nourishment for any chance to get more work done. They then make up those calories on the weekends, during business lunches, at hotels and conferences, and so on.

The problem begins by *not* eating *enough* throughout the day on a consistent basis. This is a dangerous recipe for weight gain over the years, and which is why, most of time, when I am finally able to measure someone's resting metabolic rate, and calculate calorie needs for each meal, the person is literally surprised to learn how much he or she can really eat throughout the day.

Of course, much of this surprise is related directly to the fact that most people are completely unaware of what's in the food they eat. *Dr. Shapiro's Picture Perfect Weight Loss* is an excellent resource for visuals on how different a healthy meal and an unhealthy meal can appear in quantity when you place them side by side. Healthy meals often take up two or three plates, while the unhealthy plate only takes up one.

I encourage you to purchase that book and use it as a reference. I also highly encourage you to start counting the calories in the food you eat. The life lesson you are granted will serve you forever. I do this myself about two to three times a year, and whenever else I feel a need to get back on track. For a list of my favorite tracking resources online, you can visit the website associated with this book at: www.FitnessNomadWisdom.com

What I'm talking about here has more to do with the fact that on a daily basis, you're missing too many meals, lacking the proper amounts of protein and fiber in your diet, and as a result, your metabolism is slowing down and setting you up for weight gain.

A big reason people gain weight as they continue to age is that the body's metabolism slows down. That's right, starting sometime in your thirties, your body started losing about 1 percent of bone and muscle (unless you've been performing the right kind of strength training two to three days per week all that time). As a result, your body doesn't need the same number of calories to support itself anymore. There is just not as much of you around—except for all that metabolically dead *fat*, of course.

The second reason your metabolism slows down, though, is the one I'm talking about here. When you eat poorly, and you don't eat enough during the day, your body's metabolism slows down, and starts producing more of the hormones you need to conserve fat, and crave sugar. In addition, this form of malnutrition leads to sub-optimal changes in your body's insulin and blood sugar levels. Both of which are important to stabilize if you want to get and stay lean.

That's right! Skipping breakfast or eating a high carbohydrate breakfast with little protein, missing meals, eating processed foods, not addressing post-workout nutrition, and not getting adequate amounts of protein in general will stifle your body's ability to get lean. And what will stifle your metabolism and your weight loss success most are inconsistent eating patterns throughout your day-to-day life. Ask any client of mine who has figured this out, and they will tell you that it is no longer possible for them to go more than a few hours without food. They have been retrained and have reclaimed their metabolism, their blood sugar and insulin levels have stabilized, and their physiological system is now demanding consistent nutrition. These facts ultimately keep the metabolism running at full speed more of the time.

That's what I mean when I say that you really can "Eat More and Weigh Less." Most people go through the day taking in very few calories relative to what their body truly needs hour by hour. They are on what's known as, the "Reverse Pyramid of Eating." They eat very little in the morning for breakfast and then more and more throughout the day. On most days, they never catch up. They make up for it at off times eating high calorie, low-nutrition foods, drinking alcohol, indulging in sweets, and so forth. The problem is that these eating habits wreak havoc on your metabolism and make it harder and harder for you to lose weight.

The minute you start eating the right amount of food in the form of balanced meals with adequate amounts of protein and fiber spaced strategically throughout your day, your metabolic rate will begin to increase, and your body composition will begin to change; you will begin the process of reclaiming your metabolism. Assuming that is, that the number of calories you take in is on average less than the number of calories you burn over the course of time.

Not too much less, however. It is important that on average you tip this equation by about 500 calories per day. In other words, you need to find a way to undercut the number of calories you need each day by 500 calories. Anymore, and you will find yourself way too hungry and malnourished to exercise, and unable to prevent cravings for high-glycemic index foods. Any less, and your results will stagnate and you will become frustrated. Of course, any balance in your favor less than 500 is still great. Because if you stay with this for the rest of your life as you should, then over the course of time, you will become leaner and leaner. And in my experience, the slower the process of changing your body composition, the more likely it is that you will maintain it. The more likely it is that you will have established a new way of living, instead of a short-term pursuit of superficial goals.

A note for my critics

Yes, there is still much debate about whether or not one can truly increase their metabolic rate with strength training and better nutrition. To this I have two points:

First, since I measure Resting Metabolic Rate (RMR) on a periodic basis, I can say with confidence that in a small number of cases, I have found increases in metabolic rate over time. I plan to research this fact more extensively in the coming years. I have also seen increases within the first month or two of my work with clients, when for some reason we have decided to retest RMR. It is my theory (and the premise for more study) that there is a slight tick upward of the RMR almost immediately upon commencement of an exercise program. Usually, it is offset by an increase in hunger and in turn calorie consumption, and so for the most part goes unnoticed.

Secondly, part of what I'm talking about in terms of an increased metabolic rate is the fact that when you start exercising regularly, and eating consistently balanced meals throughout the day, whether or not your metabolic rate is higher is mostly irrelevant because what's happening instead is that the metabolism is running at higher levels earlier in the day and consistently maintaining a higher rate all day long. This is likely even more important than whether or not an overall increase in metabolism has been achieved. Mostly because it helps stabilize your body's insulin and blood sugar levels, which in turn helps prevent the storage of fat.

For example, research shows that simply eating a good well-balanced breakfast with enough protein can raise your metabolic rate by as much as 25 percent and stimulate weight loss. Mostly, because it helps jump start your metabolism each day, which promotes more eating earlier in the day, and prevents that reverse pyramid of eating I was talking about a little earlier, where people eat more and more as the day goes on.

Think about it for a moment: Did you have an adequate breakfast with enough protein every morning this week? Did you eat a good, well-balanced lunch that you brought to work with you? And what about a well-balanced morning and afternoon snack? If you're like most people struggling with their weight, the answer to these questions is most likely a resounding, "No."

One hundred percent of the clients I've worked with during the last seven years, not only come in with a No answer to all these questions, but all of them who continue to struggle to get results, have more No answers to these types of questions than the clients who achieve success.

Most people, especially the women I work with, are surprised to find that their bodies need a lot more calories than they think they do every day. Of course, you aren't allowed the privilege of this judgment unless you have your resting metabolic rate measured by a professional. Something I highly encourage you to do as soon as you can. In fact, if you live in or near Madison, Wisconsin, or ever come in to town and want this test, I would be happy to provide it for you. (Go to this site for details: www.eatlikeanomad.com.)

Most of the time, people don't have this luxury. Instead, they work from predicted formulas, which are often extremely inaccurate. For example, if you predict my resting metabolic rate, you will find it to be 2,200 calories per day, when in fact, the measured number is 2,800. That's a pretty big standard error to be working against day to day. Without a measured test of your resting metabolic rate, you will likely *fail* to achieve the weight loss and body transformation goals you desire. This information is crucial in mapping out your meal plan each day and ensuring that you are taking in *enough* calories for each of your meals. If you're interested, I've compiled a series of data documenting my clients' measured resting metabolic rate as it relates to their predicted measures. The differences are astounding! You can access this data series at the same link I just shared with you (www.eatlikeanomad.com).

Eating consistently throughout the day is the key to your weight loss and body transformation success. And it isn't easy to do. It takes work, planning, and a willingness to spend some time in the kitchen preparing your own meals.

The consistent and undying theme for *all* of the clients I've worked with throughout the years who have achieved weight loss and body transformation success is the fact that they got their nutrition in order and that they continue to work at making it better *all* the time.

If you're interested in more on metabolism, meal planning, and for some recipe and meal planning examples, I have shared a ton of them at the following location: www.eatlikeanomad.com.

Your Scale is Lying to You . . .

What's the first thing the medical assistant does when you visit your doctor's office? That's right. He or she weighs you in. "Will you please remove your shoes, John? We need to get your weight."

Little by little this incomplete act has become a metaphor for a problem that now plagues most people trying to lose weight. This isn't the only act that has led to this problem, of course. There are many other suspects, including airbrushed models on the covers of magazines and worse, weight loss clinic after weight loss clinic in almost every little strip mall telling you that in order to achieve your weight loss goals, you need to starve yourself and weigh yourself on a regular basis.

Wayne Westcott, strength training researcher at Quincy College in Massachusetts, expressed the concern well at a recent lecture in Chicago that I attended. "If I could accomplish just one thing before the day I die, it would be to get doctors to measure body composition and not just weight when patients first arrive at the clinic." I mention Wayne here because he is a tremendous resource for all of us, and has done an amazing amount of top-notch research in the field of strength training and weight loss. And from this body of science-based knowledge he has written a number of excellent books on the subject—books I'll bet you've *never* heard of. No offense to Wayne, but the holy word pontificating the importance of strength training and muscle-building work seems at times to exist in another dimension—a parallel reality. I have included a list of Wayne's books at www.FitnessNomadWisdom.com.

The fact that medical clinics and your physician still haven't figured out how to more effectively monitor your body composition is a testament to the fact that as a culture, we are way behind on properly educating people about how to more effectively and healthfully lose weight. And the reason is because that measure on the scale is almost meaningless all by itself. Unless accompanied with a body composition measurement, you can be sure that *your scale is lying to you!*

Think about it this way: There are now more "diet" and "weight loss solutions" than ever before, and the weight loss industry has become a

$70 billion a year industry. So does it make any sense that we are still fatter than we've ever been as a culture? And that as a result, obesity related illnesses are at an all time high? And that for the first time in history, the younger generation may in fact end up with a shorter life-span than ours?

Something is wrong, and it has everything to do with our obsession and attachment to the scale. Your scale, on its own, is flawed technology. It truly is *lying* to you. And the reason it is lying to you is that your scale tells you *nothing* about how well you're doing to maintain your two most precious assets in life—your muscles and your bones.

Think about how long it took you to get the point where you are today. Why would you expect your body to turn itself around in a fraction of that time period? And yet almost 100 percent of the clients I work with are frustrated at the two to three-month mark in their programs because they feel they haven't lost enough weight. And I'll bet you can relate to that fact.

We have a voracious appetite in our culture for immediate gratification—the same craving that makes us fat and makes us want to believe that we can get un-fat in a matter of months. Why is that?

When clients arrive to work with me, I often spend a great deal of time in the early stages of their training and coaching programs helping them understand what it truly takes to be successful in the long run. It's one of the main reasons I wrote this book. And much of what I explain is in direct contrast to what they have been led to believe by a culture obsessed with the scale. Not only will it take time to turn your physiology around and get back to equilibrium, but you might also experience weight gain instead of weight loss early in your training program.

Blasphemy!

Especially if you've been starving yourself, knowingly or not, once you begin to feed your body the five or six balanced meals it really needs to nourish itself and sustain the work of the day, the body will begin to soak those calories in and put them back into the muscles as the stored form of carbohydrate—muscle glycogen. For every gram of muscle glycogen that you store in your body, you will store about three to four grams of water right along with it. And water is heavy. So, when you get on the scale a month after coming to work with me, and you've been working hard to train and to eat the actual number of calories your body needs to sustain itself, you are very often heavier when you stand on your scale.

Your scale cannot measure fat alone. When you step onto that evil little unassuming device inside the cozy confines of your bathroom each morning, you are *not* getting the data you need to be successful in getting and staying lean. What you are actually doing is measuring the weight of your entire body, including fat, muscle, bone, your body's organs, and all of the food and energy you have stored inside each of your cells.

Why would I even mention the "energy stored inside each of your cells?" Because it's a perfect example of how and why that enticing measurement on the scale is so misleading. And that is where all that muscle glycogen is being stored.

The stored form of carbohydrate—glycogen—is stored both in your liver and in your muscles. This energy substrate is heavy because, as I mentioned, it stores with a lot of water. As a result, the amount of glycogen (stored carbohydrate) you have in your body can dramatically affect how much you weigh on the scale each and every day. This is why low carbohydrate diets actually work to make the number on your scale go down. They cause weight loss primarily as a function of reducing the amount of glycogen, and in turn water, stored in your muscles, and in your body in general.

One of the most difficult and often potentially dismantling realities for my clients early on in their training programs is the fact that when they actually start training right, include strength training, and in turn, eat to support this effort, their muscles, which have been starving for proper nutrition, begin to gobble up the glucose and carbohydrate like a famished puppy after a long run at the dog park. All this carbohydrate gets put in those muscles so that they can recover, and be ready for more work. If you don't understand what's happening, however, when you see your weight increase, in conjunction with your new and improved exercise program, disturbing things can happen to your mind-set and your belief system about the program you've decided to implement.

"If you're doing this right," I explain to clients at this time, "You will often gain about five pounds on the scale in the early stages of your training program. As long as your body fat either stays the same or is decreasing, if even only slightly, you are making the progress you need to make on your quest for a leaner physique."

Try explaining that, however, to people who have used the scale to guide their weight loss efforts for their entire life, and what you get is often madness, disbelief, and reactions that don't serve their goals or my ego very well at all.

It's simple, really. If you stop eating carbohydrate, you store less glycogen and in turn water; on your evil little scale you appear lighter. But remember, your scale cannot differentiate between the different parts of your body.

It is for these reasons, that it remains vital for you to have your body fat measured on a regular basis and to *stop* weighing yourself without also measuring your body fat. The two pieces of data together provide extremely valuable information. Measuring weight alone, however, is like driving on a country road in a snowstorm without your headlights. Eventually, you're going to veer off the road and find yourself stuck in a snow drift.

Body composition measurements—more commonly known as "Body Fat" measurements—will provide a much more accurate assessment about the distribution of fat and lean tissue (bones, muscles, and body organs) in your body for reasons I will elaborate on elsewhere and that I've written extensively about on my blog at www.FitnessNomadReport.com. There are many ways to accomplish this measure. They include underwater weighing, use of skin calipers, bio-electrical impedance analysis (the method I currently use at my studio in Madison), ultrasound, and more. The important thing is to measure it because it's a much more accurate picture of your overall health than using your scale all by itself.

In closing this chapter, then, I would like to make a strong recommendation that you perform the following ritual—a ritual that could literally change the way an entire culture views the job of weight loss.

Go out today and buy yourself a really good sledge hammer. Take it home and set it down in your front yard. Go inside and locate that dreaded device you know as the scale. Haul that out into the front yard too. Now, make a few phone calls to friends, neighbors, and your local press and invite them over. Once they arrive, get to work on smashing that scale to pieces. Quietly sweep it up, and dump it in the garbage. Keep the sledge hammer because there are some really great exercises I can show you how to do with that. And relish in your new quest to start a whole new life, free from the shackles of your scale that can no longer tie you to it. And if you're really motivated, send me a YouTube video of your work on smashing the scale. If enough of you do it, we will have something significant to share with the world at large ☺. My YouTube username is: fitnessnomad.

So Much Talk about Diet, and No One is Talking About Muscle—

The Withering Elephant in the Room

I just finished reading the *New York Times* this morning. It's Sunday and a cool breeze is blowing through my living room window for the first time in about a week. The weather has been hot and I welcome the chance to open my windows, sip a cup of green tea, and spend some time reading the paper. I do this on my iPhone, and the computer instead of trying to fight with all of that ink and paper. The kids will be up soon and I need to be as efficient as possible so that I can steal some time to read, write, and do my research for this book.

A quick stretch following my early morning run/walk and I'm ready to get cranking. This is my favorite part of the day. I came across another article in the *Times* that was a perfect launching pad for the topic I wanted to write about this morning. It was another good article from science writer Gina Kolata. She tends to take a controversial approach in her coverage of exercise, good nutrition, and weight loss. In fact, she's written an interesting book on the subject titled, *Rethinking thin: The New Science of Weight Loss—And the Myths and Realities of Dieting.* I don't recommend the book, because I think it's full of baloney. I do think it's interesting that such a book exists, and that's what I want to talk about now.

The book itself seems to be nothing more than one 85,000-word treatise designed to satisfy those who continue to fail in their efforts to lose weight, while at the same time also helping the experts on weight loss in our country feel satisfied and justified in their attempts to lock in theories about how our DNA is to blame for all of our failed efforts. Another helpless scapegoat used in an attempt to take attention away from what is truly important—the hard work of eating strategically, building muscle, and getting fit.

What I find both interesting and disturbing in a book like this one (there are hundreds and maybe thousands of them) is the genuine and malicious pursuit of one and only one solution to our weight loss woes—dieting! In my assessment, "diet" is a four letter word, and so is "thin" by the way.

What does "thin" really mean? Think for a moment about how you think and feel when you hear the word "thin." Thin would be more appropriately used to describe Gina's discussion in her book on the subject. Her book shows that she's so scarce in her understanding of the importance of more than just eating right that it makes me hungry, but not for food.

I'm ravenous now, like a bear in the woods that hasn't eaten for weeks. My hunger has me on the hunt—on a ravenous hunt designed to chase down, capture, and devour every last one of these "experts," drag them into the gym, and show them what it feels like to use their bodies in a way that adequately takes advantage of their design. I won't let them leave until they admit that their theories about "dieting" as the panacea for all those who suffer from being overweight and obese is incomplete, like an unfinished workout, like their own pursuit of peak fitness. I won't let them leave until they spend at least six months to a year working until they can't move anymore, sweating profusely, and crying for mercy, begging me to go easier on them, and to let them off the hook for the work they should have been doing all along. This is the work they should have been doing at least two hours a week, taking a break from behind their desk, rising out of that hunching back that has become so familiar and comfortable to them. I will not rest until I have dragged them all in and had the opportunity to show them the truth—the hard, sweaty, muscular truth. Because here's the truth: "diets" don't work, muscles do! And people need to embrace the work to build them.

If this is truly where we are as a culture, and what we are willing to accept as the problem, then I want out. I want out for good, but let me take my weights with me—my kettlebells, my dumbbells and anything else that's heavy that I can carry, because I love the work. I can't get enough of it. For more than ten years, as I've battled chronic tension headaches and had to limit my activity level to some degree, I still crave it, and even though a workout sometimes means a week's worth of pain, I still do it because it feels good and my body wants its cravings satisfied, regardless of my unfortunate side-effects. That bear, that hairy man that lives inside me wants to move heavy things, climb, jump, run, sprint, and take the physiological response of the body to the limit. For no other reason than it feels good. An exhilarating rush of blood, hormones, and the ecstasy of pure oxygen reaching parts of my body that no one can see, including me. But I can feel them. I can feel them when I'm done, and I've pushed myself back from the edge I was working on—the edge of that glorious cliff that no one wants to visit because it hurts, it's too much work, and they are scared of falling over the edge to their death.

There is no reason to be afraid and it's okay if you are. You are growing, moving, and building muscle. You are growing into a new way of thinking and understanding that will set you free, like the hang glider who launches from that same cliff and with the help of the wind, lifts off and soars above, looking down in some wild combination of joy and disbelief as he or she moves farther out toward the sea and closer to the heavens. That person is in you. You are in him or her. Don't let the culture take hold of you and let you believe that you are unable to soar, unable to do the work necessary to build muscle and live your beautiful life. It is in you. I can see it in you, feel it in you, and if I can drag you into my gym, I will exorcise it out of you like a demon that you will befriend and come to behold as the most sacred creature on earth.

Diets Don't Work—People Do

The article I read in the *Times* moved along the same path as the book, and all of it makes me wonder how much Gina might be struggling with her own weight. And though that might be beside the point, if it's true, I'll have to bet it would encourage her to write more and more about the controversy of whether or not exercise really works. In fact, you can search for another article she wrote titled, "Does Exercise Really Keep us Healthy?" You can visit the following link: (http://www.nytimes.com/ref/health/healthguide/esn-exercise-ess.html).

Now, I'm not a science reporter and I have no intension of launching in to my own scientific review of the literature at the moment. I work hard instead to do the research, hone my knowledge and expertise, and then present it in a way that's easy to understand, cuts to the bottom line like a good CFO, and then outlines a specific set of systems and strategies you can put into place to solve the problem. And the problem in this case, and in general, is that no one is talking in the right way about muscle. In fact, in most of Gina's book, the word "muscle" is missing, like an absent senator. What we find instead, is more and more talk about diet, cardiovascular exercise, and how our bodies determine whether or not we lose weight. I not only find this repulsive, but I also find it irresponsible. Allow me to explain:

In the article above, the problem was identified by the author almost by accident. That's how blind we have become to what our bodies truly need. We have gotten so lost and so bogged down with the surplus of information about how we need to change our diets and start walking thirty minutes a day, that we have completely lost sight of the solution. The solution does contain aerobic exercise and good nutrition, which they discuss in detail. However, they avoid a discussion of muscle, and instead, replace it with opinions and some scientific evidence about why people are having so much difficulty losing weight.

One researcher argues that your body composition is dictated by DNA and monitored by your brain. Attempting to bypass these physiological systems is not just a matter of will power, he says. They agree that exercise and good nutrition are important, but obviously feel that they are not enough, and much of this research has been designed to reinforce beliefs that there is only so much each individual can do about his or her weight. Sadly, they are all missing the point! With so much focus on DNA, minimal amounts of aerobic exercise, and a combined ignorance and lack of focus on building muscle, you are being led to believe that there is not much you can do about those rolls that keep appearing around your waist.

The reason no one wants to talk about building muscle is that muscle is hard to build. It's true that if you're working hard, training the right way, and eating supportively, you can add one to three pounds of muscle to your body every month. In general, if you are able to add even three pounds of muscle to your body in a six-month time period, you can call it a major victory and go celebrate. But in order to accomplish that, you are going to have to put in some consistent hard work, both in the weight room and with your nutrition program. The experts think you can't do it. They believe that you're too busy or too tired or simply unwilling to make it happen. That's their problem. I believe in you, and I know what science shows us is possible. I know you can make it happen, but I also know that you are going to have to put in some serious work to do it.

The hard work you put in will not only pay off in muscle, and an improved metabolism and physique, but the accomplishment will leave you feeling stronger, empowered, and confident that you can accomplish anything you want in the gym and in your life. The experts are wrong. This is not so much about your will-power as it is about your level of discipline and a willingness to do the work that needs to be done. There will *never* be a better way to transform your metabolism, than to perform the work in the gym building muscle. This is work that is necessary to change your core physiology from the inside out. That's what this is about and in order to stimulate that change, you are going to have to work harder than you ever have in the gym, especially with the weights. Don't be intimidated by this, however, I know you can do it. I see people in my fitness studio doing things every day that they never imagined were possible. They only needed someone to believe in them. Once again, I believe in you.

Your first step is to get over you unwillingness to work at this problem. Without the hard work that's necessary to build muscle, you will not achieve the results you desire. If this scares you—good! You can't be brave if you're not scared. You can't grow and evolve as a human being if you you're not challenging yourself to perform in ways that make you feel uncomfortable. So, if you feel a little anxious right now that's okay. You have no past experience and no knowledge to guide you through something that is flying directly against what you thought you knew. It's okay, I'm here, and it's time to for you to soar.

The Experts are Actually Right About Some Things

I'm not going to spend any more time in this section of the book arguing against a growing body of research that is trying to tell you that weight loss is not only difficult, but almost impossible for some folks. For the most part, these people are doing good work, but in a limited way. What bothers me is that they are making assumptions about the human race and about people in our culture that I'm unwilling to accept. These assumptions are that we are too lazy, too busy, too limited by our DNA, and too unwilling to do the work necessary to take our bodies back—to reclaim our metabolism. And instead of being unwilling to accept this, they have chosen to cater to it, like a mom who just can't find a better way to get her child to behave than to buy him a toy every time he has a good day. Researchers are choosing to accept that people don't want to do the hard work of building muscle and transforming their physiology. I will never choose this and I don't think you should either. So, let's move on.

A Problem of Intensity

The night went dark long ago, and you find yourself already pining for spring, even though Santa hasn't arrived yet. Frost covers the lower corners of the dining room window, and you're dreading that last trip out into the back yard to let the dog out one more time. Winter has only just begun and early in December you're already wondering how you'll make it through another one.

You know that feeling, when you put your kids to bed at night in the middle of winter? The air outside is crisp and electric. The wind howls, and snow taps the windows outside. You might even have a stocking cap on to keep your head and your body just a little bit warmer. And your feet are covered with thick wool socks that you slog around in until bedtime, when you transition them into cuddling mode next to the hot water bottle at the foot of your bed underneath the sheets. The heat has been turned down for the night, and the house is bracing itself for another cold winter night, while you hope the furnace holds out for the remainder of the winter, and yet your five-year-old is emanating a fierce and vital heat that requires you to go back into her room after she has fallen asleep and remove her covers until she cools down. Even if you're on top of it and you arrive at her bedside on time, you still find that she is literally hot with sweat, life, energy, and the anabolic work of making her body and her muscles grow. She is literally an anabolic machine. Laying down new cells night after night, year after year, diligently until the work is done. You, too, can transform yourself into an anabolic machine. Just get your training right, your intensity right, your nutrition right, and you, too, will lie in bed at night basking in the heat of your anabolic potential.

The problem is that most people *never* reach their anabolic potential. Most are *never* able to get all three crucial pillars in place and working for them consistently at the same time—supportive nutrition, a solid strength training program cycled expertly over the course of the year, and regular cardiovascular exercise. Most people *never* really work hard enough, and different enough to totally unlock the human potential of their muscles. Instead, they stay below that threshold, working at lower weight, and higher repetitions, and in routines that *never* really change that much. The result is stagnation, frustration, and a body that remains in hibernation.

Up to 80 percent of your gains in muscle strength can be attributed to motor learning. This means that your body is learning to use your nervous system in a more efficient way, and the majority of your gains in strength early in your training program are due to nervous system adaptations and *not* muscle growth.

Immediately following each strength workout, your body goes to work in teaching itself how to recruit more muscle fibers to do the work the next time it's asked, and to make that recruitment even more efficient. This is both beautiful and incredibly challenging at the same time because as you become more efficient with each workout, it takes more and more effort and creativity to challenge your body effectively each time you get to the gym. In terms of building muscle, this means that in order to stimulate true growth in your muscles, you have to train hard enough to tap into that final 20 percent, and you have to organize this training in the right way EVERY time you train. If you don't, you will become another innocent victim in pursuit of elusive results for which you begin to believe there is some magic and secret formula.

The truth is, that there *is* a "magic and secret" formula, and it lies directly in two important aspects of your strength training program— intensity, and creativity. You absolutely *must* work harder, and you *must* work differently almost every time you train.

In my two decades of experience as a fitness coach, I can tell you that in 100 percent of the clients I've worked with, this has been the number one problem. Either they are not performing or never have performed any strength training as part of their exercise routine, or they have *never* really worked hard enough to tap in to that final 20 percent of their potential.

A brief history lesson will help shed some light on this subject.

Strength Gains Take Hard Work

"Hard work is when someone asks you to do something you really don't want to do, and you do it anyway"

—George Carlin

I love that quote because when it comes to strength training, I would say that most people really don't want to do it. In fact, they often work even harder to avoid it, make excuses for why they can't do it, and ultimately grow old and frail at a young age. That's unfortunate.

"Wow, I've never worked this hard before!" is a statement I hear very often from clients when they begin their work with me. The comment usually comes from those who have been exercising on their own, tried some strength training, tried eating better, and have yet to see those elusive results showing up underneath their shirts. I love it when that happens, because it tells me that we are going to see some big changes now that they're working hard enough (assuming, of course, that they can stay with it for the long run.)

Another woman from my boot camp was at the studio just the other day. She attends one of the morning boot camp classes in addition to the ones I hold at a local school gymnasium where I have very little equipment to work with, and where we use a lot of body weight exercises to provide the resistance. "I never even considered the bottom rack," she said.

She was referring to the bottom row of the dumbbell rack where the weights of the dumbbells start at thirty pounds, and move to the right in five pounds increments until they hit sixty. Although I know people generally don't work hard enough when working with weights, this still sometimes surprises me and catches me off guard like a third base coach who in an instant is playing a game of dodge ball for his life as he attempts to avoid the foul ball that he barely saw coming his way. "How could you simply *never* consider the bottom rack?" I thought. Well, that is What this Chapter is All About

Make No Mistake, This Stuff is Hard Work

When the idea of weight lifting (which I will refer to throughout the book as strength training) started to find its way from the world of the body builder and the power lifters in the Olympics into the mainstream, the journey was clunky, awkward, and has meandered, like a five-year-old who just removed his training wheels, ever since. For the most part, we stayed on course, but along the way, we've fallen down, scraped our knees, and every once in awhile we've bumped our heads really hard. Thank goodness for our helmets. Two problems have arisen from this evolution. I will reveal them here.

The first problem actually leads us to the second:

In an effort to oversimplify the work of bodybuilding and powerlifting for the rest of us, no one was quite sure how to separate the specific objectives of bodybuilders and Olympic athletes, and the objectives of the average folks at the office who suddenly notice that they need a new belt, or that their pants might rip when they bend over to retrieve the paperclip just dropped on the floor. No one considered that even these people, still need to work hard at the gym building muscle. They might not desire the physique seen on muscle beaches in Los Angeles, but what they do desire is a pair of pants that won't rip, a belt that fits them comfortably, and a bathing suit they can wear with pride. And in order to have these important things, they still need to build muscle. So, oversimplifying their program is not only an insult to their capabilities as human beings, but also an irresponsible attempt at a solution to their problems.

Any mere mortal would love to believe you when you tell him or her that it's not necessary to work that hard to see muscles grow. Why do you think you can always find an eight-minute solution on a Saturday afternoon infomercial? People want to believe it's true.

Another great example of this first problem is others who have made the irresponsible effort to cater to those women who are afraid they might "bulk-up" from too much resistance training. I cover this in more detail in another chapter. Many women are afraid of building muscles because they have been led to believe it is unattractive, unfeminine and an embarrassing manifestation of their insides coming out for all the world to gawk at. Ridiculous!

Much of this has been driven by scary images of women bodybuilders who look like they jumped out of a comic book. And images of women who have not only used the magic of extra testosterone in the form of steroids to help their bodies grow abnormally, but who have also trained for many hours a day to get their muscles to respond in this manner. This is a very different scenario than the average woman who simply wants to train two to three days per week, build some muscle, rev up her metabolism, and get home in time to prepare some fish tacos, feed her family, check her e-mail, prepare for another day at the office, and go to bed feeling rested, energized, and full of the vitality she deserves.

In an effort to cater to this fear (and that's all it is—fear) you will find resistance training programs that do not include the right combination of strength and growth work to stimulate true and lasting muscle growth. In its place you find "Cardio Pump" classes and many derivatives that include programs and classes full of high repetitions and low loads that are great for helping you stay fit and build aerobic conditioning, but that render the muscles of the body unwilling to adapt, grow, strengthen, and produce the kind of muscle-building results your body needs.

Remember, it is muscle growth that makes all the difference for your long-term success in getting and staying lean. Your furnace needs to be stoked, and you need to work harder to manifest the flames. In fact, you will most likely need to work harder than you ever have, and lift weights you never imagined lifting. You will have to take a brave and conscious journey down onto that second rack of the dumbbells, where the muscles will be made to grow like one-year-old oak trees alone in the country. Year after year, laying down more mass, widening, and digging down into the earth to settle their roots, becoming more beautiful, full, and shapely with each passing year, and ultimately, ready and now prepared to last another fifty years.

The second problem relates to the first in that yes, people seeking general fitness have different needs than a bodybuilder or Olympic power lifter, but to oversimplify and ignore the important and body-altering scientific methods and techniques that these individuals use to build muscle and strength is one of the most important mistakes the fitness industry has made to date. Deciding that the average person seeking "general fitness" (a problematic term itself), should get an oversimplified version of what we know works is irresponsible, ignorant, and frankly insulting. The result is that both women and men come to work with me and discover immediately how ready their bodies are to respond to their training when asked to perform the right kind of work at the right times, and with the right amount of progressive overload and progression.

No one should make the mistake of blindly adopting a strengthening and conditioning program because it was presented well in a magazine article, used by a successful weight-trained athlete, or billed as *the* program that will get *you* the results you are looking for in twelve weeks or less. This is a lifelong body of work that takes patience, expertise, commitment, discipline, and most importantly, a structure and design that takes advantage of scientific principles about how the body adapts, builds muscle, and gets stronger, and at the same time makes plenty of room for you, your individual body structure, physiology, psychology, and life challenges. If you don't have all of those important ingredients, you will create a lifelong struggle with your body, your weight gain, and your peace of mind.

There is no one best way to train, and at the same time there are scientific principles that should guide your training throughout the year. Void of this structure, your body will revolt in disgust. Much in the same way you most likely revolt in disgust when you see a picture of yourself on the beach from your last vacation, or every time you look at your aging and seemingly helpless physique in the mirror after you get out of the shower every morning and weigh yourself.

This is your time now—your time to grow roots, widen, ground yourself, and build the most beautiful body you've ever had in your life, one ring at a time, one rep at a time, and one season of strength and growth at a time.

Some Final Notes About The Hard Work

Remember, you'll find many books and strategies on the subject of building a better body and achieving lasting results for your weight loss, and the creation of the body you've always wanted. There is just one problem in all the books, DVDs, magazines, and monologues. They make me think of a dried up banana peel sitting on the side of the road in the hot burning sun in August—sitting there rotting, conforming to the earth, and making its way back into the soil, recycled, composted, and soon just another drift of soil on the shoulder of the road.

Many of the books have good information. I've referred to a few of them for research in writing this one. And they all contain one very common theme, or I should say lack of the tough idea I'm writing about in this section of the book. There really is no "magic" solution. You just have to do the work, and do it regularly. And four times a year, you really have to pound it, like one of those bodybuilders who passed down this right to us. It is our job and our responsibility to carry it forward, like the Olympic torch, burning in the hearts, minds, and bodies and into our eternity. Our evolution depends on this and hence our bodies do.

I can hear your concerns and complaints already. They're like a far away voice coming from the other side of that dark tunnel you walked down one day and didn't even notice—the tunnel that took you to where you are in your life right now. You are fatter than you want to be, out of shape, and wondering how in the hell it all happened. Your story unfolded in that dark tunnel when you had your blinders on and couldn't see. You simply thought it was dark more than it should be but that was part of life, the way things were. "You're getting older now honey, you should just accept it, move on, and join the rest of us here at the other end. It's not so bad here. Mediocrity is easy and a lot less work. We never have to confront any of our demons, face any of our fears, or go into the light and challenge our souls to do all those things that feel so uncomfortable. All we have to do is ignore that tunnel we passed through and forget about how beautiful that orange and red light looks from this end. How beautiful that woman's voice is who sings in there to the tune of that bowl she strokes. We can't really hear that any more anyway. The television is on, the kids are screaming, dinner still needs to be made, and I need a nap—just a quick nap so that I can forget about having to think about what it might be like to make my journey back through that tunnel and to that place I once knew, where my body cooperated with me and where I felt so much vitality, and life in me every day. I don't think I can make it there. I'm too weak, I'm too tired, I'm too afraid. And I don't want to do the work. Come over here with us honey, we'll take care of you—"

"No, I won't! I will stay and fight! I will do my part to build the legend! I will face my fear, and ignorance like a warrior—a peaceful warrior who fights with openness, knowledge, and surrender." I will work with the kind of surrender that allows her to let the work pass through her like spirit moving in the room—a spirit that's been with her all along, begging to guide her if she would only let her; a spirit so present now that goose bumps travel up the nape of her neck and make her feel a little chilled and exhilarated all at the same time; a force that makes her want to move, work, and go into the light of her physiology, tap into the work her genes have been waiting for, and build glorious muscle with the best of them. This is a journey that will bring out the best in her, and all those who come in contact with her as her adventure unfolds. And every time she considers the possibility that she might not be able to do the work, stick with the swirling smoke of pain and pleasure that wrap around her, she will wait for that spirit in the darkness of the tunnel until it pushes her forward. No matter how afraid, or unsure, she will trust that force working behind her, let it pass through her when needed, and dig for it when it seems to have been lost. And as long as she stays connected to that spirit of this legend, she will have the all the courage she needs to sing with the woman at the other side of the tunnel where the light is so beautiful, so orange and red at the same time, that it will lift her up like a catapult and bring her that much closer to the heavens.

Let go of your concerns now and let the work take hold. Surrender to the beast of your resistance, and surrender, surrender. There is so much work to be done.

It's easy for me to get excited about strength training and building muscle. I've been doing it my entire life. Even as a young kid, tearing up the playground, I was connected with the body's desire to move, adapt, and become stronger and more fit. I remember going to sleep at night and thinking that it was such an inconvenience that I had to spend all this time resting. I couldn't wait to wake up and run again, swim again, and ride my bike to the race track again. I was (and still am) intimately connected with my body's need for physical movement on a daily basis, and while I don't race around on the BMX track anymore, I spend time doing a lot of other things that most people avoid.

As I just discussed previously, one of the most important forms of exercise that the majority of people avoid is strength training. Sad, but true, only about 20 percent of regular exercisers are engaged in this form of training, and it's one of the main reasons you're wearing out and getting fat as you age. Strength training creates an intimate connection between your body and your brain—a connection that cannot be built any other way, a connection that even the best walking program could *never* excite.

I certainly don't want to take anything away from you. Walking is a great form of exercise and activity and I do a ton of it myself. But it is not enough to bring your neural connections out of hibernation—a hibernation that leaves your body weak, frail, and metabolically stagnant.

Following are my Top 5 Reasons Why Walking is Not Enough Exercise

Walking won't wake you up. Even though it feels like you're contracting 100 percent of each muscle involved in walking, you're actually only engaging about 10 percent of your muscle cells when you walk on a level surface. Walking up a hill increases this to about 30 percent, but that is it. Your body is very efficient and because the muscle cells at work are evenly distributed throughout your muscles, your body can survive with only a 10 percent engagement of muscle tissue. The rest of you is just going along for the ride. Another way to look at it is that your body is literally so efficient that when you walk, it distributes the work from one motor unit to the next so that the same group of muscles is only working every third step or so. Great if you're Forest Gump and trying to walk or run all the way across America. Not so great if you're simply trying to get fit in forty-five minutes a day.

Walking Cannot Wake Your Fast-Twitch Muscle Fibers. Your muscles have strength and endurance fibers and they are each very different. They are also known as your fast twitch (Type II) and slow twitch (Type I) muscle fibers. When you walk, your fast twitch fibers almost never work, and these are the fibers you really need to stimulate for muscle growth and to rev up your metabolism. Walking won't rev them up.

As a side note, I've recently discovered some research showing that slow-twitch fibers grow, too, when asked to perform very specific types of strength-training protocols. I simply wanted you to know this for now, and will plan to cover it in *The Fitness Nomad's Book of Wisdom, Volume 2.* ☺

Walking Doesn't Damage Muscle Cells. At first, this might seem like a good thing, but I want you to make a distinction here. There is a difference between damage to your muscle cells and damage to actual muscle tissue, bones, or joints. When you exercise, you *must* create *cellular* damage in your muscles so that your body is forced to recover. If you don't do this, it's like coasting downhill all the time on your bike. It's a lot of fun, the wind feels good on your face, you get a little rush, but you could do it all day long without stopping, and your body is not forced to recover and regenerate stronger tissue and stronger physiological systems. Walking never really creates the kind of fatigue you need to stimulate the kind of muscle damage you need to adapt and build muscle, get stronger, younger, and more fit.

Walking Doesn't Build Muscle. For all of the reasons above and more, walking doesn't build muscle. And you need to build muscle, or at least maintain what you have to stave off aging, rev up your metabolism for weight loss, and draw out your potential—the true potential of your physical presence in the world.

Walking Doesn't do Much to Stimulate Bone Growth or Maintain Strong Bones. Aside from some possible miniscule changes in bone density in your hip and heel, walking does NOTHING to help you maintain your bones as you age. If you're interested and you visit the special website devoted to this book, you will find a story about how one woman was completely misled by her doctor and what happened to her bones as a result. (See www.FitnessNomadWisdom.com.)

Be Coachable

I'm Your Coach—You Don't Always Have to Love Me or Even Like Me.

One of the great challenges of this work is that it's decisively personal. You get stuck in your life, don't feel good, gain a lot of weight, get sick, watch your energy level drop through the ground, and you call me, willingly.

In the beginning, it's exciting! A new place to play. The exercise feels good, lasting, and refreshing. New bonds are formed; everyone grows and as long as you are achieving good things, life and your pursuit of peak health are bountiful. And then, it happens—

You get stuck. Your feet won't move. Your arms are tired. You want a beer. You want to "skip this one." You miss an appointment. You let your life creep back in. All of the old belief systems, emotional sticking points, and bad habits are suddenly back, and if you could only find someone to pin it on, then you could just move forward. Only there's no one to pin it on, because it's all about *you*. And boy is that scary! So scary, in fact, that when your coach begins the work of attempting to nudge you, challenge you, and help you leap these obstacles, he or she no longer seems like your best friend. He or she is the enemy. Or at least it seems that way, when your coach pushes you into such uncomfortable places where no one else is willing to send you. It's no fun to like him or her anymore. This is where the true work and growth happens, however, if you're willing to stay.

Unfortunately, this is also where so many walk away, disgusted, mad, and unwilling to take a closer look inward. That's because on the outside there's always another coach, another gym, another excuse to justify your limitations. And in the end, you can almost always find good company there. The people there will let you get away with your denial, and with you being a coward.

Now before you go coming after me again, let me share something very important with you:

I'm not perfect either, but I also don't expect less from myself just because it's so much easier. Let's face it—the growth is pretty damn uncomfortable at times. I've had chronic pain for more than ten years that almost no one knows about because I don't like sharing it. I don't want any excuses for being less productive as a human being. I don't want your sympathy, that's such a weak position. What I really want is for the pain to subside. I could accomplish so much more.

There's the rub, though. The pain is there for a reason, so when I'm fully grounded, I embrace it instead and I let it teach me about life, compassion, and steadfast determination. I let it teach me about patience and empathy for others with similar afflictions. And I use it to make me stronger when I wake up in the morning and I feel as if I might vomit before I get dressed. It goes away and I move forward. I take the next step and I grow.

Three years ago my sister died, and a year later I gave up alcohol for good because it had helped kill her. Alcoholism is a bad disease. I choose life and being present instead. This is a personal choice that was difficult and so much more for the better. I grew a lot from that one. And to be clear, I was never an alcoholic, but it runs in my family like a silent infection. Heck, it runs in our culture like a silent infection.

I opened a business just ahead of one of the worst economies my lifetime has ever seen. I'm here all the time and I think about it *all* the time. I don't sleep well because of it. I feel sick sometimes because of it. And I still come in, ready (most of the time), to coach you; to be with you, and to dance in this existence we call life because that's what this is all about—being present, responsible, and fully willing to take ownership of who you are as a human being and everything that is possible for you to accomplish, if you will only let go of your inhibitions.

If you will only let go of your rationalizations and your justifications, you will begin to see a life on the other side of that wall—obstacle—that is a place where the grass really is greener. You will have to fertilize that grass to make it grow, though. You can't have a beautiful lawn if you never feed it, and put your intention directly into its roots. You can't just expect that weeds will never grow, and that someone else will come along and cut it for you when needed. You have to do it yourself, and you won't always want to. And that is where you will learn the most about yourself.

Deep inside the core of who you really are as a human, is a sense of peace like no other—the peace of knowing that the *resistance* is where all growth truly happens, the peace of knowing that no one is perfect, and that no one has it all figured out. This is the peace of knowing what I know, which is that as long as you stay grounded and true to that peace that lives within you, you will grow, evolve, and fulfill your ultimate mission as a human being.

Yes, I know you think you come here for exercise and good nutrition. But in truth, those only provide the foundation for the true and lasting work that until now, only a select few have chosen.

What will you choose?

The Big Three

I talk all the time about the fact that we have no shortage for information on health, fitness, and weight loss. There are so many books, magazines, and shows on the subject that you could keep yourself busy full-time trying to keep up with all of the advice. This book is no exception—it adds to the list, though I hope in a different way. I hope it leads in a way that begins the journey back from all the confusion because there exists great potential for this abundance of information to confuse the public. Especially when you don't have a guide—a fitness Sherpa to help you find the easiest and most effective path up the side of the mountain because there really is no "magic" solution. I've already said it, but it's worth repeating: you just have to do the work, and do it regularly. And four times a year, you really have to pound it, like one of those body builders who passed down this right to us. You don't have to build the same kind of body they do, you just have to build some muscle. It is your job and your responsibility to do your job and carry this forward as you would the Olympic torch, burning in the hearts, minds, and bodies of humankind. Our evolution as a species depends on it.

Most people fail in their attempt to carry this right forward. They fail in their attempts to take control of their bodies in order to get fit and lose weight. They fail for many reasons, but at the root of the problem is their lack of follow-through. And their lack of follow-through is a direct result of three very important problems that need to be addressed. In the same way a golfer must address the ball with precision before every single shot, you too must address these problems one by one. Otherwise, you will always have trouble finding the fairway and the green. And there will *never* be that glorious victory party late in the afternoon at the club house—you wearing your RED shirt.

Here are what I call THE BIG 3 PROBLEMS

First, void of an accountability system to keep you on track in pursuit of your goals, you have no one person, process, or system in place to ensure that you keep going. Everyone runs into obstacles along the way. They cannot be avoided. They are a catalyst for your growth. Most of the time, we need a coach and support system in place to help navigate them.

Second, in spite of the endless stream of solutions you find without even looking that hard, people continue to struggle to get fit and get results because they lack the expertise necessary to adapt these solutions to their own physiology, psychology, and individuality. Too often, I talk with people who are frustrated because they've "tried, but nothing seems to work."

The fact is that in *all* of these cases where I'm talking to someone who truly believes he or she has "tried everything," there is *always* something missing. In all of these cases, it is evident to me that these people have implemented the wrong system at the wrong time, and remain unable to see the problems with the system they have implemented. Most importantly, they have failed to take that "magic system" they decided to "try" and formulate a plan—a plan that should include specific goals and a specific program design that will get results. Most people begin their pursuit of peak health without much of a plan in place and very little, if any, expert guidance. Those two facts, combined with the lack of a system for accountability, almost always leaves them meandering, like that kid on a bike who has just removed the training wheels.

The third part of this "Big 3" is the importance of having a solid structure in place that will provide you the support you need to be successful. This support can come in many forms, and you will have to figure out what you need personally; but trying to go it alone is difficult and just plain lonely. Finding a community of people, including a coach, who understand the journey you have embarked upon, and who can share your experience, who will understand your struggles, and keep you inspired, is one of the most important discoveries you will need to make as you begin. This community will provide many things along the way that your spouse, your friends and colleagues, and your kids cannot. One reason is an unconditional acceptance of you. You have decided to do this because it is important to you. They will not judge or threaten to undermine your progress. They will only want to share with you along the way so that all of you can accomplish far more than you ever thought possible.

Failure to address these three important problems—lack of accountability, lack of expert guidance, and a lack of support—leads directly to failure because the pursuit is incomplete and ultimately leads to a lack of follow-through. Inevitably people reach a point where results don't manifest quickly enough, results cease to exist altogether, or boredom and other life challenges and responsibilities settle in like an unwanted house guest you feel you should tolerate because he or she is family.

When people don't follow through, they feel as if they've failed. And they have, but only because they failed to address these three very important problems, and as a result, follow-through was impossible. The most important one of these Big 3 is the expert guidance. That is what leads people to victory—their coach. In the end, instead of seeing the problem for what it is, people too often blame themselves, give up hope, and abandon any belief that the hard work of exercise and good nutrition really does work.

Lacking this expert guidance, designed to ensure that you are building muscle, would be like trying to burn a campfire without any wood. Those twigs, leaves, and scrawny little branches you've collected instead might burn for a few minutes or so, but they'll never last long enough for you to keep yourself warm and toasty at night.

Building muscle takes time, hard work, and special attention to the details of your strength training program. The work also takes courage, care, understanding of yourself and the process, and faith in the science that stands behind it. The work requires you to exit your comfort zone in the gym, head toward the back door, ignore the "Emergency Exit Only" signs, set off the alarms, and run toward your freedom from all that you once believed was true.

In order to push open that door and break through every last barrier standing in your way, you will need accountability, expert guidance, and support. Your long-term success demands your attention to these three very important problems. The Big Three as I have named them here.

Remember, this sense of failure that you are currently holding is false. You are only missing the hidden recipe for success. Your sense of failure is based on your current belief that what you have been doing, or have done in the past, was the right formula. When the truth is that for every single person I've *ever* talked with about reaching their health, fitness, and weight loss goals, not one of them came to me with all three of the Big 3 squared away.

The result is a sense of failure that is based on a creaky foundation, because you never quite had the right formula for success. This is somewhat like building your house on the San Andreas Fault. Eventually, those plates are going to move, your house is going to tear in half, and you will either fall into the center of the Earth, or move quickly to the side of your house that feels the most safe, and not come out for a while. You might consider rebuilding, but not on that fault again. You will need to find more solid ground, or at least different ground. And if your house has fallen in on you more than once, if you've failed to achieve the results you're after more than a few times, it is natural that you will begin to wonder whether or not the Earth holds any ground that is solid enough for you to live safely upon.

Eventually you end up in that little red chair in my office, realizing finally that you can't avoid the hard work, that you need a good coach with a proven system to guide you, and that the foundation you need is bedrock, not sand, gravel, and volatile plates that move in the desert heat. You will find this bedrock in the on-going support that a good coach, his expertise, and his team and fellow clients and colleagues can provide for you. This is a house of people and experts that can help you build, follow-through, and face your fear, demons, and misconceptions. Because otherwise, you will be lost forever, found only thousands of years later when those plates have finally broken apart, California has sunken into the ocean, and your frail and over fat physique washes up on the shore and they study you for clues about how a race of people forgot how to thrive on good nutrition, movement, and a lifetime physical work ethic.

I Feel A Little Bit Beefy

Misconceptions, Myths, and Mystical Beliefs About Muscle: Where Women Often Go Wrong

The following story helps illustrate what I would consider the second most common problem when it comes to an individual's struggle to get fit and lose weight.

"I feel a little beefy!" she exclaimed as she walked through the entrance to my fitness studio lobby. (I will call her Allison for the purpose of this story because I know how serious it would be for any woman to be publicly identified as "too beefy.") That would be a catastrophe bigger than your grandma's thighs. Girls don't want to get "big and bulky." They want to "tone," "sculpt," and "shape" their bodies. They want to carve out the contours of their muscles as if they are being made a sculpture by one of our time's most gifted artists.

"I'm trusting you," she cautioned, "because I have to tell you, it's freaking me out!"

I try calming her down with the usual techniques and the trusted knowledge and experience that I possess. For me, what Allison is experiencing is a sign that all of the hard work she is performing is paying off. The system is working and she is building muscle. Yet, she continues to fret a little (sometimes a lot), and though I know she doesn't believe me completely, she moves toward the workout floor and begins her warm-up on the treadmill.

One of the reasons she is freaking out is that her scale is telling her that she weighs an additional five pounds. That evil little device that sits on her bathroom floor taunts her like a bully and has betrayed her again this morning. That five pounds she dropped initially when she first began her program about a month ago has returned and then some, and not only that, she feels "beefy," too. There must be something wrong. "John must be a quack." The entire program has fallen apart and somehow the scale has been granted the authority to tell her so.

"Stop!" I say. "All of this is a sign of progress, and all of this is simply a sign of your misconceptions about how to build muscle, why it's so vital to your long-term weight loss success, and why so many women quit before they have even begun to carve away the clay and begin the journey of making fine art of their bodies."

It's no surprise, really. Considering the mountains of misinformation that exist and the ill-guided perceptions in our culture about what truly makes your body the healthy, fit, and the energized machine that it is. No, it is really no surprise that women react in this manner. And it's okay. You didn't know. No one told you, and in fact you have all been led to believe that your scale and your high repetition cardio pump workouts and body sculpting classes are the answer. I'm here to tell you that they're not, at least not all by themselves. And I'm here to explain how these myths came to exist, and why they're bogus! Stay calm, warm up, and prepare yourself for the true and lasting work that your body will need to endure and solidify your place in the legend—a legend built one woman at a time.

One hard and bursting workout at a time, you will stimulate your body to grow, relish in changes that you do not recognize, and finally understand what all those men are doing in that special section of the gym that you thought required a certain amount of testosterone to enter.

Here are the top five misconceptions women have about muscle:

Women believe that the purpose of lifting weight is to tone, sculpt, and shape their muscles. Big mistake! The truth is that the purpose of strength training is to build muscle. And in doing so, your muscles will become more toned and you will bring out their natural and normal shape (determined primarily by your DNA). The problem with the false concepts of "toning, shaping, and sculpting" is that women often pursue these ghosts with routines that contain a lot of high repetition, low weight exercises. The theory is that this will produce the desired result without making the muscles too "bulky." The problem is that you can't tone, shape, and sculpt muscles that you haven't built yet, and when you're doing all that high repetition stuff that you perform during those "cardio pump" and "chisel" classes, you're not building muscle. Instead, you're building endurance in the muscles you already do have. That's not bad, and it *is* a start, but it's not what you're looking for. Really. It's true.

As a result of this first misconception, **women believe that high repetitions and low weights are the way to success.** As I pointed out above, this type of routine only builds endurance in your body and in your muscles. It *will not* build muscle. And though you might feel like progress is being made because you are burning some extra fat and drawing a little more of your existing muscle into view, you will not produce the results you're after in the long run unless you cycle your strength training program and start lifting a lot more weight at least four times a year, which brings me to the next point.

Women fear that lifting too much weight is going to make them huge, and unattractive, and as if they will start growing hair on their chest. (Well, okay, that last one is a stretch.) But If I had a buck for every time I've heard from a woman who is afraid she is getting too "beefy" or "bulky" I could buy a lot more kettlebells and rent a separate room for them.

True, women and men increase muscle and strength at roughly the same rate in the same training programs, but let me explain something to you. A very typical result from proper training would be that after six months to a year of lifting lots of heavy weight, the typical man or woman would be lucky to build even five to six pounds of muscle. Now, for just a moment, imagine that a baseball literally represents the size of about one pound of muscle. Even if you were able to build five to six new baseballs, they are not all going to stack up on top of your shoulders or in your butt. They are going to spread out nicely all over your newly "toned" physique and in truth, you'll only notice that your clothes fit better and that you look that much more fantastic in your swimsuit. In addition, while this is happening, you will also drop a proportionately greater number of pounds of fat. Now, if you imagine a cantaloupe representing the size of one pound of fat, and you lose twice as many fat pounds along the way, it is very hard for me to believe that you are actually going to look *bigger* as a result of your strength training program. Not to mention that those pounds of baseball are so much more firm and compacted. I think we can all agree that pounds of muscle would be preferred over pounds of fat. They're sexier, more metabolically active, and make you a lot stronger than the cantaloupe.

Most Women Believe That Aerobic Exercise is The Answer to Their Weight Loss Goals. Endurance exercise is part of the equation, but not the panacea it often becomes for fat loss. True, if you are only looking at the workout itself, a 140-pound woman will burn an estimated 512 calories running a twelve-minute mile pace for an hour. Keep in mind that this also includes the one hundred or so calories you would burn at rest whether you were running or not. An hour of serious strength training will burn about 25 percent less, say about 384 calories. But here's what everyone always misses, "The controversial Afterburn!" The fact that when you're activating more of your physiology and building muscle in the right ways, your body is burning more calories *all day long.* In addition, I would still highly encourage you to do the cardiovascular work. In fact, you *must* if you want results. But you also *must* perform the strength work to help maintain the integrity of your joints, your muscles, and your body in general if you want it to hold up under the demands from all this training.

Intensity is the most important factor for your post-workout metabolism (your "Afterburn"). All that hard work you put in at the weight room will work for you all day long and well into the night while you're sleeping, hunting down fat cells and eating them alive like that rabbit in your garden who likes to destroy your strawberry patch. Serious strength training signals your body to burn higher percentages of fat at rest. And that's crucial to your long-term success. **In one study, both women and men were burning 22 percent more fat for energy fifteen hours following a serious strength training workout.** The researchers in this study concluded that the exercisers would have needed to burn twice as many calories during their aerobic workout—eight hundred, instead of four hundred—to reach the level of post-workout fat oxidation achieved by the weight-lifters. That's a dedicated soldier working for you all day long, and all you have to do is perform some really serious muscle building work, two to three days per week. And four times a year, this work needs to be focused even more on strength and muscle building. Remember, your body, your future, and our legend as a human race depends on it.

Unfortunately, many women (especially middle-aged and older women) believe that building muscle is for men only, or for younger people only . . . Hopefully by now, you can see that this is ridiculous. And that by building muscle, you are cultivating two of life's most pure and essential assets—your muscles and your bones. No longer should you be afraid that the wrong things are going to happen to your body, that you can't do the work you need to do to make muscles grow, and that you might end up looking like one of those crazy women in *Muscle and Fitness* magazine who has used extra hormones in the form of testosterone to make her body grow in unique and deformed ways.

You will now take charge, lift more weight, and take proper care of your muscles and bones. This will build strength not only in your body, but also in your heart and mind, where it will travel out like a disciple, inspire others, and move even more women to do their part to solidify the legend.

If you are interested in a short YouTube video I recorded to clearly demonstrate the difference between one pound of muscle and one pound of fat, go right now to the resources page I've created for this book at: www.FitnessNomadWisdom.com.

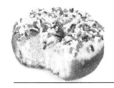

CHAPTER THREE

WHAT IS STRENGTH?

Your Strength Endures as Legend—

You Must Fight!

Building strength and stimulating growth in your muscles is on-going, never-ending—a timeless project that builds the legend of humankind.

Sound daunting? Good, that means you're growing—not just growing muscle, but growing as a human being.

One day I was working out in my fitness studio. Working on this thing called muscle, my assets. The experience was thrilling. Yes, thrilling. The feeling of moving heavy iron and weight through the atmosphere, around in space, up and down, and through my body is cleansing, like taking a hot bath from the inside out.

At one point, I asked Kirk, one of the trainers who worked for me at the time, for a spot on the bench press and I realized something very important—something I know instinctively, yet I believe it still needs to be reinforced. No matter how hard you've worked, or how tired your body might feel, there is always more work and more growth possible. All you have to do is ask.

"How many are you doing?" Kirk asked.

"Not more than five," I replied. I then proceeded to lift the bar from the rack, my feet in the air—core, and trunk engaged like a lion on the hunt—and began moving the weight up and down.

"Good!" Kirk encouraged at just the right time. "Strong, breathe. Inhale" (as the bar moved down), "breathe" (as I pushed the bar up).

When I reached the down-stroke of rep number five, I was on my way to a job well done.

"Okay, keep going," Kirk encouraged.

And I did, and only because he asked me to and I agreed in an instant that more was possible. The set ended with eight repetitions and the last two were like a fog rolling into the San Francisco Bay, mysterious and sudden and numbing in a good way—a soft, cool blanket that is refreshing in its surprise.

Kirk wanted me to do nine, and though possible, I was already finished in my mind. As I reflected on the experience, I decided that if I had stayed strong in my head, one more (possibly with a little help from Kirk) would have been possible. I say "strong in my mind" because that strength reaches out to the rest of the body like an old friend after a year of absence.

I've heard another say that strength can endure like a legend, even beyond our lifetime. I think this is true because there's something that happens when you go into that fog of the work—that misty place where almost anything is possible, like the growth of the legendary bean stalk into the clouds. It's that place where time stands still and once and for all your body takes on its own agenda, an agenda that exists beyond conscious thought, somewhere deep in the DNA where your physiology cries out for more because that's what it is built for.

You can't buy it or borrow it. You can only cultivate your body's innate willingness to build it, like the mastermind behind the skyscraper that almost seems to erect itself. The vision of what your body needs and craves is always present. When we ground ourselves in the kiva and hold heavy things until our muscles burn in delight, we tap into that vision that is lying dormant in our DNA, hiding from us—that vision our Creator had for us all along to be strong, pursue our evolution like dynamos, and build a better and stronger body as a foundation.

To build this kind of strength, you need patience, understanding, and self-love. You can't let your head and the thoughts that build storms there, hinder your progress and infect your DNA with the virus of weakness that only exists when you are not grounded enough to feel the truth digging deep into the earth from your feet. Building strength and muscle does not come quickly and your work is never done because the work of your evolution is never done.

Overnight strength is mirage, a trick of the body's neurological system, a quick adaptation designed to allow you to accomplish more—if you're willing to perform the work and dig the trenches. Eighty percent of your strength gains at any one given time are primarily a result of the increased efficiency of your neurological system—more efficient recruitment of motor units that innervate your muscles and ask them to contract. This is an exquisite process and a symbol of the universal plan for all of us to evolve, grow, and be strong. This is the human body in the heat of the work it was designed to do all along. We simply lost touch with this truth in our cubicles and sedentary lives along the way, attempting to find solace in Dilbert, when instead we should have been looking for it in that gym downstairs. The one the wellness committee built for us a year ago and that no one is using.

This adaptation of the nervous system is important because it helps us build the foundation we need to keep going, keep working, and ultimately keep growing muscle. Yet, it will only happen if we are working hard enough and often enough to feed the roots.

Staying in those high repetition ranges where the weight is light and the fog is thin, if present at all is nice. What we really need to do is conquer the fear that comes with the thicker fog—the one that only allows us to see a few feet ahead of us. A fog that forces us to trust the work and ourselves and that allows us to believe that lifting more weight is not only possible, but thrilling. Like the foghorn under your feet on the Golden Gate Bridge.

Lifting more weight is also essential to stimulate muscle growth. If 80 percent of your gains in muscle strength can be attributed to motor learning, this means that 80 percent of your strength gains are due primarily to your nervous system's ability to recruit muscle fibers that were not previously being used, and learning to use those fibers in more efficient ways.

This is good news for all aspects of your training and fitness, but it is also the same reason that most people often hit those dreaded plateaus where they experience diminishing returns for the time they spend at the gym. Especially women who tend to lift in higher repetition ranges and with lighter weights, muscle gets stronger (to a point), especially early in a training program. If a new and more significant stimulus is not applied, however, it begins to lie dormant, like a hidden treasure at the bottom of the sea. Only a brave and well-planned exploration can dig it up.

This exploration is your willingness to start training your muscles in a new and much more challenging way, at least four times a year. Unless you do, you will continue to experience less and less return on your investment of time, and soon will find yourself wondering why you decided to do this work in the first place.

Your exploration will take you on a search for the treasure that is waiting for you deep in the belly of every one of your muscles. Those cells and your DNA have been waiting for you to begin digging—to begin the journey of unlocking the codes that will stimulate your muscles to grow. Your muscles will grow, like a tulip in early spring, moving first a little slow as the ground continues to warm, poking its head cautiously above the earth. And then, as the sun shines and it is fed, it too taps into the roots of its DNA and the resulting photosynthesis allows it to grow toward the sky, bloom, and provide leadership for the rest of spring.

Your muscles hold those same codes, those same memories from other lifetimes where gladiators tapped in to the source and used it to fight until their death. Like it or not, you too are fighting until your death in a different way. Like it or not your muscles and bones will either grow or die and once you hit the age of thirty to forty, they begin that process of death and wearing out. But they won't if you fight like the warrior in the coliseum—not if you fight.

You must first fight to unlock the potential of your muscles. You must cut through the fog and break down your cubicle like that warrior entering the stadium. Break yourself free from the shackles that have been tied to your ankles by a culture's move away from the physical activity and work that our DNA demands. Then, you must fight every day for the work your muscles desire in the gym—the work that stimulates their growth, your growth, and the strength of you and the world as legend.

The Wonders of Strength:
When muscles get Stronger, You Realize Your Full Potential

It is my goal in this book to leave out as many "shoulds" as possible. I think the last thing we need is another expert telling us what we "should" do. You can go to the bookstore and find a hundred other books on either side of mine that will do that for us. Many of them have great information, but I don't approach my training and coaching that way with clients, and I don't want to approach this book that way either.

What I would like to do is make a compelling argument for what I'm talking about here. And what I'm talking about in this book is the importance of building strength and muscles in your body. More specifically, the importance of doing serious strength and muscle building exercise at least four times a year. I'm not saying you don't need to train all year long. I'm saying that you need to break up this training on a quarterly basis and really hit it hard, stimulate those muscles to grow, and then get back to the next phase of your training program.

So, in the spirit of inspiring you instead of lecturing you, this next section of the book outlines what I call the Wonders of Strength—all the big benefits of doing strength training. Many of these benefits are happening quietly inside your body and providing you with the engine of healthy and fit aging that everyone desires.

Personally, I'm only forty-three years old—relatively young, but seasoned enough to realize how important this process is for healthy aging. I'm smart enough to realize that my body will not last forever, and that I can't just hide from the facts. And the facts tell us that our bodies will lose about .3 to .5 percent of bone mass starting at age thirty if we're not careful. And our muscle tissue will go at an even higher rate, so that by the time you get to be eighty (if you're lucky enough to make it that far), you've lost approximately 45 percent of your bones and muscles. This is a process that started when you weren't looking, in your thirties, and then just kept wearing you out because you never did anything about it. It doesn't have to be this way.

Muscles are the Engine of Your Youth

Stronger muscles positively affect ten key biomarkers for aging. These biomarkers include the following:

- Muscle mass
- Strength
- Basal metabolic rate
- Body fat percentage
- Aerobic capacity
- Blood glucose tolerance
- Cholesterol
- Blood pressure
- Bone density
- The ability to regulate body temperature

You need to develop lean body weight that makes you active, fit, and energized. Flabbiness and fatness is not an inevitability of the aging process. It is an inevitability of being sedentary and slothful.

There's no question that we all lose peak fitness as we continue to age. The good news is that you can do something about it. You do not actually build new muscle cells when you do strength training and build muscle. In fact, as you age, you continue to lose muscle cells at a rate that depends directly on what you are doing to offset the loss.

When you are building muscle, what you are actually doing is adding mass inside each remaining cell, which is packed with protein—the red meat. Fortunately, the potential for growth in your muscle cells that remain is outstanding. So, before you throw up your hands and submit to the aging process, let's get to work on taking advantage of what you still have available. If you get to work and keep at it, you really can thrive into your sixties, seventies, and eighties, and beyond.

The exquisite nature of the human body allows you to literally lose half of your muscle and still end up stronger at eighty then you were at twenty. Sound like a pretty good deal? I think so.

Strength Builds a Strong Foundation for Your Body and Your Life

Chances are good that you've likely heard this before—muscle is active tissue that works for you at rest. Building and maintaining more of it will increase your metabolism, help you burn more calories, and ultimately help you achieve the weight loss results that you desire. In addition, muscle strength and growth also builds a stronger and more efficient body that allows you to live your life the way you want to, compete the way you desire, and prevent the wearing out I mentioned above.

Improvement in energy level is one of the first true signs that you have activated muscle tissue in a new and exciting way. You can see that fact in many of the Nomad Victories listed at the beginning of this book. Remember that muscle tissue is a lot more active metabolically than fat tissue. Because it burns about three times more calories per day than fat, it takes more work for the body to keep it going. This work leaves you feeling awake, alive, and stronger than you were the day before.

Strength builds a foundation for your training program and for those four times a year when you are really going to hit the gym hard, build more muscle, and in turn experience even more benefit. This is a lifelong process, and if you are consistently focused four times a year building strength and, in turn, muscle in the body, you will build a stronger and stronger foundation for your life, your fitness, your competition, your next training phase, and whatever else you want to accomplish in your life.

Strength work also builds bone and helps you maintain all of your connective tissue like ligaments, tendons, and cartilage so that every time you train and every year that passes by, you continue to lay down and maintain the bedrock of your body and your life.

Muscles Shape You Smaller

Many women in particular worry that strength training is going to "bulk them up." As I pointed out earlier, the truth is that one pound of muscle is about the size of a baseball and one pound of fat the size of a cantaloupe. Which one do you think provides more bulk? As a woman, you also don't have enough testosterone to get big and bulky without steroids. Only about one in one hundred women have to really be concerned about that. And even then, the question is more about your belief system than avoiding a very positive reaction of your body.

Fat also accumulates wherever it wants to, while you can lay down muscle at your discretion by working a well-rounded strength training program for your total body. And if there happens to be an area you would like to place more emphasis, you can go for it!

Muscle Makes Your Scale Irrelevant

Most people I meet, and almost all of the ones I work with as a fitness professional and coach, have an unhealthy relationship with their scale. My advice to them, and to all of you, is that unless your scale can measure your body fat at the same time, toss it into the woods. Muscle weighs more than fat. So, when you're strength training, the scale can't tell you what's happening to your body composition. And as your body composition changes, which is to say that as you gain lean muscles and rid yourself of that unhealthy unwanted fat, the scale won't move as much as you think it should. In fact, when you follow the six-month training system I've designed, which has the primary goal of helping you take back your physiology, very often, not much happens on that scale early in your training program. It's not until months four through six that you really begin to see the fat melting away. Fat liberation is everyone's favorite stage, but it takes time to get there. And for the full details on that training system, you can visit the website I've created to support this book located at www.FitnessNomadWisdom.com.

During the first season of strength and growth, you will often see your weight increasing, and though I encourage people to stay away from the scale during this stage, they often ignore my advice. As a result, much of the coaching I do early in my work with people is in helping them understand that they need to change their relationship with their scale. This is often difficult but only until people realize how irrelevant the scale becomes when muscle is being built.

Here is a Good Example of What I'm Referring To

Lolly is a client I worked with in the past. Following nine months of training and eating right, she had lost only fifteen pounds. In nine months of grueling work, she only lost fifteen pounds on the scale. Most people would consider this a complete disaster, and often do, which leads to their abandonment of belief about whether or not strength training, regular aerobic exercise, and supportive nutrition actually work.

Along with Lolly's loss of fifteen pounds, however, came a loss of fifteen inches in all parts of her body, and a 5 percent loss of body fat. This is true and lasting body composition change at its best. Imagine it this way: she lost 5 percent of her total body weight in fat. That equates to about eleven pounds of fat lost. She dropped eleven cantaloupes from the inside of her body. And as a result she will tell you with passion now about how she has never felt better and about the fact that though she has achieved this scale weight before, she has never fit into her clothes the way she does now.

Now, if she had been relying on the scale completely on her own with no one to help her build muscle and truly understand what was happening to her body along the way, it is likely that what seemed like insignificant changes along the way might have derailed her.

Unfortunately, this story repeats itself over and over again in people's lives and instead of sticking with the program and gaining a true understanding of what it takes to transform their physiology and their body composition, they give up. Lolly's video story can be found by visiting the "Success Stories" tab on The Fitness Nomad website at: www.TheFitnessNomad.com.

Muscle is Money in the Bank

It takes time to build assets in life. Often it takes a lifetime. The same is true with building muscle, one of life's most precious assets. Your muscle is also an asset that won't fluctuate with the market. The only way you lose it or weaken its position is by a lack of action, work, and follow-through to continue to build and maintain it. What if all you had to do to make sure your retirement plan was safe from the economy was get to the gym for an hour a day? Would you do it?

What if you started looking at the muscle in your body as a true and lasting asset? What might that allow you to consider? Your muscles are your secret retirement plan—the one that will make all the money you've earned and saved worth spending and worth living for.

Every pound of your muscle burns thirty-five to fifty more calories per day, and without any added effort. Now, let me head you off at the pass of those destructive thoughts that start filtering through your mind at the moment you contemplate the seemingly meager thirty-five to fifty calories per pound of muscle. Let me put that into perspective. For every pound of muscle you lay down, you have it working for you to burn those extra calories. Yes, it takes a lot of hard work to lay down and build one pound of muscle, but once it's there and you are working to maintain it, it begins working for you for the rest of your life, just like Apple stock. This is often a new way of considering how the work in the gym pays off for you—a new and essential way to shift your belief system because this really is about the rest of your life.

Go down to the bookstore today and peruse the shelf and you will see what I'm talking about. Almost any book you pick up and read about strength training has an eight-week or a twelve-week or a sixteen-week program you can follow for massive results. It just doesn't work that way. Yes, if you work those programs and they are designed properly, you will get results, but the idea that eight to sixteen weeks is all you need is misleading, irresponsible, and contributing to society's misconception about how important it is to build muscle in the body all year long, every year. And about how important it is to focus your strength and muscle building at least four times a year.

If every pound of muscle equals your ability to burn thirty-five to fifty more calories per day, and without any added effort, this means that during the course of a year, you will burn up to an additional 18,250 calories for every extra pound of muscle you lay down. That totals about five pounds of fat burned for every year you keep that muscle intact—every year for the rest of your life! That's the kind of work that leads to true and lasting body transformation. That's the kind of work that builds life's most precious asset. Let's put as much of that in the bank as possible shall we? I'm headed down to the studio right now to make a deposit. I would love it for you to join me. Here's why.

Ten pounds of lean muscle added equals 180,000 extra calories in a year. That would help you burn fifty-two pounds of fat! But to build those ten pounds we need to get to work, and stay at work. We're building your retirement plan here. And unless you're putting in the time, no one else is contributing to your 401K. So, get up from that chair, give me a call, and let's get to the studio. I'll see you there! Don't live locally? Find a good coach in your local neighborhood, or take advantage of all the great resources I have waiting for you at: www.FitnessNomadWisdom.com

Strength and Muscle Enhance and Prolong Life

"Aerobic exercise saves your life; strength training makes it worth living."

—Henry Lodge, MD
in *Younger Next Year*

I just finished watching my sixty-nine-year-old mother-in-law put on her farm boots so she could till the garden. It was a prophetic image. The struggle to bend over into bones that are breaking apart and muscles that have been neglected for years was hard for me to watch. It also struck a fair amount of fear into my own bones as I witnessed her struggling to don that second boot, which kept flopping over, causing her to lose her balance repeatedly. I was afraid she was going to fall.

My wife, Laura, and I have been encouraging her for years to start doing some regular strength training. Even fifteen minutes a day would likely change her life dramatically. I've seen it happen over and over again. Give a sixty-five-year-old unfit individual some chair squats to perform a few times a day and you will have a friend for life! The strength in their legs alone is life-altering. And of course, they are not just building strength in their legs when they perform a squat. Any compound movement like the squat requires an exquisite coordination of millions of muscles cells, nerves, tendons, and ligaments, all performing their part at just the right time and with just the right amount of force.

Strength training builds muscle, and that's what this book is about. But there is also a hidden network of changes taking place behind those curtains that are as important to your long-term fitness, health, and success as those shoulders you have noticed emerging from underneath your shirts. These neurological changes are paramount and provide the foundation for continued strength training, all forms of movement, prevention of falls as you get older, and ultimately to your living into your seventies without having to worry about struggling to put your boots on.

Strength training enhances this elaborate network of nerves that link your brain and muscles. The problem is that no one is really aware of all of these changes that are taking place deep inside the body. We aren't aware of the nerve decay that is taking place in there. It's not like your teeth that get x-rayed and checked by your dentist once or twice a year. Nerves decay largely unnoticed. And this decay is the main reason that your joints wear out, your muscles get sloppy and uncoordinated, and your ability to be the spirited young person you used to know fades into the corn field.

The casual motion of daily life is not enough to turn your body on, and regular strength training and the manufacturing of muscle tissue can change all that.

For an even more detailed explanation of the physiology and how regular strength training and muscle growth can make you younger, visit www.FitnessNomadWisdom.com.

The Science of Strength

Don't let this section scare you or turn you off from moving forward. And don't skip it either. I know that if I heard someone say he or she was going to talk about, "the science of strength," I might just turn right around and get back to what I was doing. My intention here is to put it in perspective because, until you have at least a basic understanding of what strength in your muscles and your body actually is, we cannot move forward.

Now, you and I know that when we feel stronger, we feel empowered. But unless you're a fitness professional like me, you have likely not taken any time to contemplate what is actually happening in your body to create this.

What does being Stronger Actually Mean?

This knowledge is likely to change your perspective forever. It's like being in the room when your first-born child is about to arrive. The feeling is exhausting, electric, and exhilarating all at the same time. Then, suddenly, life changes forever.

There are many reasons that people avoid the gym and exercise in general. Most of them are nonsense when you get right down to it. Simply a lot of denial wrapped up in a tight little sack that no one wants to open—a package that arrives daily, and that no one wants to sign for at the door. Denial is a topic for my next book so I will leave it at that for now.

I believe one of the biggest reasons people avoid the work that is at the center of building strength and muscle is a strong blend of discomfort, and a reality that people often don't want to go inward and exorcise the demons. There exists both conflict and opportunity in this discomfort, and it takes a well-trained mind to stay in it long enough to let the outcomes speak for themselves. And when I say "long enough," I mean working long enough in each set to challenge your body, long enough in weeks to work the system, and long enough to last a lifetime. That takes discipline, presence, and steadfast pursuit. Let's face it, on any given day, you have personal choices. First, you have the choice of whether or not to *ever* get started and second, a choice of two types of mind-sets at the gym. You can make the choice that makes ten pounds feel like a hundred, or one hundred pounds feel like five. You choose.

As a quick anecdotal side-note, I can tell you from firsthand experience over the last two decades as a personal trainer and fitness coach, that when I have a client who complains about every set and how hard it is, I have a client who won't last very long unless he or she chooses to reset his or her mind—a client willing to change his or her belief system.

Building strength breeds a type of wisdom in the body that can only come when you go down into that deep dark cave and light a fire, sit with it for a long while, and wait out the fear, discomfort, and anxiety about whether or not you are choosing to evolve. You will likely hear sounds and hear voices in the dark parts of that cave—audible remnants from ancient times. Some of them will call you deeper while others will encourage you to throw sand on that fire and walk away. Brave souls move deeper, even when there is no light, because brave souls know that the ground they stand on, the winds in that tunnel, and the voices they can only faintly hear are the ones they should be listening to, in spite of their trepidation.

Defining Strength

Okay, let's get this out of the way and make it quick, because the other stuff is more fun to write and quite frankly, though it's important for you to understand what is happening physiologically, there are much more important metaphysical aspects that you need to connect with to make this happen.

Strength is the ability of a muscle to exert force. More specifically, it's the maximum amount of force a muscle or muscle group can generate through a specific movement pattern. The ability for you to grab those thirty-five or forty pound dumbbells, one for each hand, and then proceed to squat up and down repeatedly. This feeling makes your body feel as though it's being pulled into the earth. And as you move them upward, it's a feeling that makes you feel powerful, challenged, and asking serious questions of yourself about how many you can actually do. Most importantly, to build primarily strength in your muscles, you need to lift a weight that does not allow you to do more than ten repetitions, and that ideally fatigues you somewhere between the fourth and sixth repetition. Have you ever really done that? If so, well done. If not, you really are in for a treat. But we will get into more of that later. For now, we're just talking about the science of strength.

Going back to that first sentence in the last paragraph I want you to pay close attention to one phrase, "the maximum amount of force" that a muscle can generate. Put even more specifically, strength is built using "maximum voluntary muscular contractions."

It's easy for your eyes to glaze over when you start reading stuff like that. I can attest that in research for this book, I was excited to get back into the science and the books and all of the great stuff there is to read and study on the subject, but even at times I feel a little overwhelmed with all of the scientific language.

The point I want to emphasize is "maximal" because that is the missing ingredient in almost every client I've ever worked with, consulted with, or even just conversed with on the subject of their training programs. The work has to be a "maximal" challenge to the muscle, and in turn, to the physiology that is working within its belly. If it isn't, true and lasting strength is *not* built, muscles *don't* grow, fat is *not* burned, and people don't get results. Then one day you read an irresponsible article in *The New York Times,* and if you're not careful you are led to believe that all this hard work doesn't work anyway. Visit the www.FitnessNomadWisdom for a full video explanation of this article I referred to here. Trust me, it does work, it's just that the work has to be "maximal" and you have to have the three pillars I talk about in the problem section of this book firmly in place at all times. I explain in more detail elsewhere in this book and on my blog about how and why you need to train maximally. For now, I only want you to plant that phrase into your inner conscious mind so that it can get to work on the importance of how hard you need to work to get results.

One more important concept I should at least mention here, however, is that of **Progressive Overload**. The reason I want to mention it here is just in case you don't read the rest of the book. A lack of **Progressive Overload** is probably the number one reason people plateau and stop getting results. The number one reason a place like Curves stops working for you after awhile.

Progressive Overload refers to the importance of continually increasing the workload (stress) placed on the muscles as they become stronger. If you get stronger, and you don't change the stimulus, nothing more will happen. It's like not watering your plants in the middle of summer when it isn't raining.

If you don't get the progressive overload right, your work is like your garden—producing for you for a few years, and then nothing. It provides full, ripe tomatoes and strawberries out of the ground until one summer nothing happens. Your plants and patches wilt, and fruit is missing from the vines because the crop was never rotated, the ground was never fertilized. You forgot, you didn't know, or you simply ignored it.

For now, remember this: to build strength and ultimately stimulate growth in your muscles, you need to lift an amount of weight equivalent to 75 to 80 percent of your maximum effort. Once again, can you really say that you have ever done that, or that you are doing that regularly? Because, once again, I can tell you from my own personal experience as a fitness coach, that most people are not.

If Toning is Your Goal, Strength is the Method

"I really just want to tone up." I've probably heard that goal expressed a thousand times in my fitness career. And it's okay because that's one of the big reasons people decide they're willing to start doing some strength training. Their skin is not hanging on them as it used to. It's dripping off the bottom of their arm where their triceps used to reside. Their chest droops underneath their t-shirt, and bounces up and down when they run. Their thighs rub together constantly, and their belly shakes like a cooled bowl of Jello almost any time it detects movement. All of this makes them want to tie a sweatshirt around their bottom, and wear loose-fitting clothes all the time. And never mind that swimsuit, they simply decide to avoid the pool. Better to live in hiding than face up to the drooping and aging physique.

Eventually for some, however, their drooping physique becomes unacceptable, at least initially, or at least at the point where they actually look at themselves in a picture from that vacation in Hawaii. "Could that really be me?" They ask themselves. So they embark on the journey of making it different, and quickly learn that a quick fix is out of the question, and that void of the expert guidance of a coach and trainer, it is difficult to get the balance of strength training, cardiovascular exercise, and supportive nutrition just right. By the time folks reach the red chair that they sit in at my office for a consultation, they have tried all of the other options that exist with little or no lasting result. They finally decide to ask for help—at least a few of them anyway.

There are recurring themes in everything I hear from prospective clients, and one in particular that tops the list: "I want to tone up."

"Of course you do," I say. But that's not really the point. The idea of "toning up" is alive, like a living breathing Big Foot in the woods. Invisible to the average observer, yet commonplace in all of those beautiful young women you see in *Shape* magazine demonstrating the "toning" routines you see in the articles you might even have stacked on your nightstand at home right now.

While the idea of "toning up" is pleasing and seems plausible, it is actually a false pretense. The concept sounds cool when written in a magazine or book, but it lacks any tangible and definable meaning. It's another good example of the misinformation that gets passed down from one fitness enthusiast to the other, like a sacred ring that no one knows was originally purchased on State Street downtown from some guy with only one tooth. Why does this happen?

The strength work that your muscles do is mostly done without the immediate presence of oxygen. This is known to us physiologists as anaerobic work, and you have probably heard the term before. The term "muscle tone" refers to your muscles' readiness to perform physical work. It is an electrophysiological phenomenon that reflects the ionic flow across muscle cell membranes. Strong and fit muscles have more of this flow and as a result are more toned and ready for action.

Lack of exercise, especially strength training, makes you weak, and that creates drooping muscles directly as a result of the fact that you're not asking them to do anything. Those triceps you're hiding underneath all of those long sleeve shirts are begging for you to ask them to exert force, move heavy things, and do some serious physical work. If you neglect to feed them, however, they begin to droop in protest and will never return again to that upright and attentive position that you lost in the woods while searching for Big Foot.

Aerobic exercise (with oxygen) like running, biking, or swimming improves tone a little bit, and you may notice slight differences in the way your body looks with this type of exercise, especially in the muscles you are using for the specific activity. An example is in your legs if you're cycling. But strength training and strength building is what truly improves muscle tone—the more intense the better. Once again, that's why it's essential for you to, at least four times a year, spend time building strength and growing your muscles. They are begging for it, and so are your sleeveless shirts!

The truth is that "muscle tone" is simply a by-product of strength training work—a nice fringe benefit of muscles that are now being asked to work in a very specific way, and are growing stronger and bigger as a result. Increasing your metabolism, stimulating bone to grow, and recreating you as the energetic person full of prowess that you thought you'd lost touch with long ago. "Muscle tone" as a primary goal is just another example of how we all get caught up in pursuing this work for the wrong reasons.

Even more problematic is that most of those exercise programs in those magazines sitting on your bedside table that claim to improve "muscle tone" are really low-intensity aerobic strength-training programs (lower weights and higher reps) masquerading as the kind of muscle-building anaerobic strength work that truly increases muscle strength, size, and tone. If you want to get tone, you need to be strong, and the only way to get strong is to train much harder for that strength at least four times a year, and beyond.

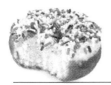

CHAPTER FOUR

WHY DO I WANT MORE MUSCLE?

Introduction

The Vital Importance of Building Muscle at Least Four Times a Year

There is one extremely important topic that I'm covering with gusto in this book that is somehow missing from so many other discussions—The sheer and lasting importance for building strength and stimulating growth in your muscles. In fact, you're probably tired of hearing about it by now. If so, good. I have discussed many other topics that are important as well, but this topic is top on the list. My focus on this one very important concept is important because it is most likely missing in your personal fitness regimen. It is also missing in an accurate and meaningful way from most other books, magazines, journals, fitness studios, gyms, and wherever else you might go searching when you're looking to beef up your knowledge about how to train, get fit, lose weight, and build a better body.

If you find that as you're reading this book, the questions are coming faster than you can keep up with, good—keep reading! Write those questions down, but keep reading because chances are that those questions are coming from the fact that I'm asking you to think in an entirely new way about your current health and fitness routine. Once you finish this book, you will have an entirely new understanding, not only of the importance of building muscle, but about why so many people fail to lose weight. And you will be "armed" with the information and knowledge about how and why it is of great importance that you build strength and stimulate growth in your muscles. And if you have questions you need answers to, I encourage you to post them on my Facebook page at: www.facebook.com /fitnessnomadreport. I *will* answer them.

Personally, I'm frustrated with what I see on the shelf at the book store anymore. And it's not that the information is bad or even inaccurate. It is simply missing a vital ingredient that is keeping you from what you really want to achieve in your body and in your life. They're not doing it on purpose, and no one is attempting to mislead you. Well, some are, but that's another story. The point is that all of it is making things more complicated than they need to be for you. And many of those authors lack the experience I've had over the last two decades working directly with people who have been down these roads, opened those rusty gates, and walked down the path into the meadow only to find that the trees had all been cut down long ago. The information they received about what they would find there (if they find it all) is old, outdated, and lacking that vital ingredient I mentioned earlier—muscle-building information.

By the time someone sits down in the red chair in my office to tell me their story about how and why they got here, and how they've failed to achieve lasting results, they are almost ready to give up for good. They've been to the gym (at least on occasion), bought the books, been to Weight Watchers, worked with trainers, and tried LA Weight Loss with early success that dies like a fading sunset drowning in the ocean. And here they sit, in the same body, with the same expression, the same disbelief, the same reluctance, the same problems, and the same questions about what makes my program so different.

So I'll put it to you once more before we get started—Muscle! You know what muscle is. I know what muscle is, and the entire world talks and publishes daily more and more information about why muscle is so important. And yet no one has given you the road map for success. No one has been able to sit you down on the bench press, hand you an amount of weight you've never even considered before (making you a little nervous), and walked you back into that meadow where the trees have been replanted, the prairie grass is growing tall, and everything is full of life again. It's that place where you can now begin to build your most important asset possible in life—Muscle! Muscle is an asset more valuable than any stock option, bucket of gold, or house on a hill—an asset that represents the bedrock of your entire existence.

I want to show you why it's so vital, and why so many have failed and missed it in the past. So pay attention, sit up straight, and get ready to change the way you think about muscle and life forever.

Aerobic Exercise Is Not The Answer

Too Much of it Will Actually Make You Fatter

When most people begin to feel the effects of extra fat accumulation beneath their skin, in their bellies and thighs, and in all other areas of the body in which it loves to congregate, they decide to do something about it, at least for a short period of time. And one of the great fall-backs for most people is aerobic exercise like running, swimming, biking, rowing, and so forth.

Often, people will find some early success, and sometimes this success is too much for their own good. Here's a great example: A woman I worked with for a short period of time said she had lost more than eighty pounds by eating well and walking every day. She walked *every* day—rain or shine, snow or ice, and in wind chills cold enough to make your nose fall right off. But a couple of years later, half of that weight is back and she is afraid that all of her hard work is going south for the winter. It is—unless she starts building muscle.

This is what I mean when I say that early results with aerobic exercise can really hurt people in the long run because they don't realize that without the necessary muscle-building exercise along the way, they are setting themselves up for long-term failure and frustration. They will likely lose even more lean tissue along the way, and prevent continued results in the form of weight loss because aerobic exercise is more about enduring than long-term muscle building. Relying on aerobic exercise exclusively is like making a fire without any slow-burning wood or coal—burning the fire with only lighter fluid to sustain the glow. For a short period of time, the fire will burn very bright and hot, but it won't sustain itself for hours on end as it does when you have some good, solid, thick wood to burn. You know—the way it smolders into the night while you sleep in your tent when camping.

When you lose weight, you lose three things: water, fat, and sometimes a little bit of muscle. When you avoid strength work and muscle-building activity, you lose a lot of muscle tissue. And this is disastrous. Strength exercise builds muscle and that stokes the furnace, keeps your metabolism running hot, and provides the foundation for all your work. In fact, a good, solid strength-training program improves your ability to perform even more intense aerobic exercise, which burns more calories in the long run. But you can't rely on aerobic exercise alone.

Aerobic exercise is an all-time favorite because it's easy to implement: You put on that old pair of sneakers from the back of the closet and go for a run. You join a gym and hop on a treadmill. Any monkey can do it. It makes me think of the people I see at the gym all the time. I'm thinking of one young girl in particular who walks for endless amounts of time on a treadmill. I warm-up, do a little walking on the treadmill myself, get my strength work done, take a steam and a shower, and then head out to pick up my kids from the day care center and she's still there, walking on that treadmill. Let me explain briefly why this is so disastrous for her and why it will ultimately make her fatter.

Let's say our hypothetical subject is a two-hundred-pound person. (The girl I'm referring to at my gym by the way is not 200 pounds. She's petite, young, and beautiful and what I like to call a "skinny fat person.") At the same time, our hypothetical subject is missing important prime-time years in her life where she could be building muscle. Not only will this catch up with her as she continues to age, but she's wasting a lot of valuable time on the damn treadmill, staring into the television that sits on top of it, and surely wondering why her body just won't "tone up" more.

Okay, back to our two-hundred-pound person who eats two thousand calories per day and doesn't yet exercise. For her New Year's resolution, she has decided she will commit to waking at 5:30 every morning and drag herself to the gym, even in the dark morning sky of Wisconsin, where it is almost always easier to stay in bed on a December morning than wake early and leave the house. Thank goodness for that indoor parking at the gym she joined, and for her attached garage. She can actually jump from one location to the other without having to go outside. I wish I had that luxury.

She decides that in order to drop the extra sixty pounds she's been collecting over the years, she will start exercising aerobically hard enough to burn about three hundred calories per day and at the same time will eat about three hundred calories less per day so that now she is consuming seventeen hundred calories per day instead of two thousand and burning an extra three hundred, which in turn creates a solid six hundred calorie deficit each day. A reasonable plan in most respects, although it's missing one key component. Can you guess what it is?

The journey begins and she is proud to report that in spite of a few mornings each week where she really has to fight with herself to rise and move toward that gym, she has done it. Three months later, the sun is starting to show its face when she pulls out of the driveway. She feels more energized; colleagues have noticed small changes she started feeling in her body after her first month of training and progress is being made. "Why didn't I start doing this a year ago?" she asks herself.

In her first three months she loses fifteen pounds and drops her body weight to 185. Not bad—significant improvement in three months" time. Not the one to two pounds per week of weight loss she read was possible in one of her magazines, but still, progress. And she feels so good. What a bonus. She doesn't realize, however, that she is about to reach the end of the road—that dreaded place so many people reach at this stage of their fitness program when strength training and muscle-building exercise is missing.

She'll drive out onto that mesa one morning, look across the canyon, and wonder how in the world she will reach the other side with no bridge and no path to follow. She'll drive around on the mesa for awhile, looking for a crossing, a path through the canyon, or maybe an invisible bridge that will magically appear if she keeps coming and searching the plateau day after day.

The search itself will keep her busy enough and interested enough, for awhile, to keep going, keep searching. After all, this mesa is a lot higher than the one she started on four months ago. The air is cleaner, birds sing a little louder, and she can see for many more miles around than she could before. In fact, her car even seems to run better at this altitude. Everything in her life has improved. If only she could find that bridge.

Physiologically her body, though it feels good and has dropped some extra weight, is stagnating. And now, to continue her weight loss momentum, she has three choices, and only two of which she can see. She can cut her calories even lower to say fifteen hundred per day or increase her time on the treadmill at the gym from forty-five to sixty minutes per day. Or, she can do both. In thinking this through, she becomes concerned because she is still forty-five pounds away from her weight loss goal. How far is she going to have to cut her calories to make it there and how much more aerobic exercise is she going to have to perform each day? It's already difficult for her to get to work on time, and she is certainly not going to get up any earlier. Not only that, but spring and summer are approaching and she knows that many more distractions are waiting for her as the warmer seasons approach.

Can you see what's happening here? Without the necessary muscle-building exercise, this poor woman is going to continue to cut her calories until she can't take it anymore, and at the same time she is going to attempt an increase in her aerobic exercise (if she can find the time). In addition to this being difficult for her to do, it will also put the body into starvation mode where her blood sugar is running too low on a regular basis, and does not have the nutrients it needs to rebuild after all her aerobic exercise. It soon will begin calling to her for more food.

Weight loss (at a much slower relative pace) will continue to come for another short period of time until once again, fifteen hundred calories and sixty minutes of work on the treadmill will only be enough to sustain her current body weight, but not stimulate any more weight loss. The cycle will continue for as long as she can stand it, which is usually not much longer, and then she will throw her hands in the air. Summer will arrive and she will decide that she's just one of those people with a slow metabolism. And she will be right. She just doesn't realize that her slow metabolism is her own fault.

Remember that I mentioned earlier: when you lose weight you lose three things? Those three things are Fat, Water, and if you're not careful—MUSCLE! At this point, this woman will begin losing muscle—her most precious life asset. More valuable than the house she just purchased (you know, the one with the attached garage), the diamond ring her husband will buy for her one day, and the trust her grandmother will turn over to her, when she dies. You get the picture.

Why does this happen? Well, in order to lose weight, you have to create a caloric deficit in the body. In other words, you need to burn more than you take in on a consistent basis. That's the big secret, okay? It's the secret that everyone wants you to believe they have the ultimate answer to. It's energy in and energy out and that's the bottom line, well . . . sort of.

Yes, you have to cut calories a little bit and then you have to get to work burning more, but if you're not careful, and you don't do it just right, you create a deficit that is too large and your body's physiology stops cooperating. This is mostly, because your central nervous system needs glucose to survive, and in order for your body to shed fat, your insulin levels must remain stabilized. And when you cut your calories too sharply, and your blood sugar drops, you're not only hungrier than you need to be, but your insulin level is no longer stable, and your body has to go looking for sugar anywhere else it can find it. Unfortunately, for you—the person cutting corners on your calorie consumption and the need for strength training—the body can get that glucose from a couple of the amino acids in your muscle tissue. This is an efficient survival mechanism, because it actually accomplishes thee things.

First, it provides the sugar the body and central nervous system need to survive.

Second, less muscle tissue means less of that active metabolic tissue that the body has to support.

Third, your body can survive a lot longer with less muscle around.

So, by continuing to perform that run you keep taking on the treadmill every day, and combining that with a severe cut in calories, you end up wasting away into a literal bag of bones. And even your bones and joints begin to feel the problem eventually, because one of the primary ways that bones grow is through the muscles and tendons that tug on them. Less muscle equals less tugging and less bone growth and maintenance. Maybe we should call the woman in the story a bag of skin instead.

Most people don't realize any of this is happening, of course, because they are obsessed with the scale in their bathroom—the one that sits next to the toilet. They must mount it day after day to reinforce all of the hard work they are putting in at 5:30 in the morning. And if they're losing heavy bone and muscle tissue, that number on the scale moves down nicely. Life is good until you drive out onto that mesa where there's no bridge, no hiking trail, and seemingly no way out except back to where you came from. That is the place where all hope is lost. Where all your exercising and dieting don't work, and that infomercial you watched last Saturday while you walked on the treadmill at the gym starts to sound pretty good. All of those before and after pictures are compelling, after all, especially since the dial on your scale has stopped moving and you have found yourself in the land of the lost or at least the land of the un-knowing.

Your body is a precision instrument designed to adapt to your needs minute by minute—a mechanism designed to take you through life like a warrior if you train it right. When you begin to starve yourself in the manner described above, your body goes to work right away releasing two hormones that aren't in your favor, somewhat like that neighbor's dog who likes to hop your fence and poop in your yard. You end up with a lot of unnecessary cleanup to do unless you build a bigger, stronger, and impenetrable fence.

Lipoprotein lipase is one of those hormones and this one tells your body to hold on to its fat stores. When you cut calories too steeply, your body thinks it's starving and that precision instrument goes to work immediately. This is one of the reasons it's so important to have that after-workout shake every time you train, by the way. Because if you don't, you will undermine the work you just did, because now your blood sugar is low. The body goes to work releasing very important enzymes that will help facilitate rapid uptake of glucose back into your muscles cells, but not if you don't feed it. If you don't feed it, you miss the opportunity and your body breaks down muscle to get the sugar it needs.

The second critical hormone released by the body in this dire physiological situation you have created with too much aerobic exercise and too few calories is cortisol. Cortisol is a stress hormone that you want to prevent from circulating in your body as much as possible. Stress hormones like cortisol promote fat weight stored in the belly (to help preserve energy for starvation). These stress hormones also promote sugar cravings because sugar, my friend, is the quickest and easiest form of energy for the body to utilize. That's one of the reasons when you're "dieting" you have so much trouble staying away from sweets.

The result of all this is a body that is now programming itself to hold on to fat stores, break down muscle tissue, and force you to eat sugar to survive. Not a great combination for the typical bohemian athlete who is already sitting around too much anyway. In fact, it's a great recipe for weight gain in the form of fat. It's a great recipe for a lifetime of struggle with your weight, your body, and your ability to age like a champion.

Pull Back the Curtains

What if I told you that probably the only things standing between you and fifteen to twenty pounds of weight loss are your muscles? Would you believe me? Do you have any idea what I'm talking about? Are you curious? I hope so, because this topic is very interesting and for all of the clients I work with, muscle is the difference-maker in their fitness program. In fact, building strength and muscle in the right ways at the right times of the year is the difference-maker for most bohemian athletes. And if you're curious about what I mean by "bohemian athlete" you'll find an explanation on the resources page associated with this book at www.FitnessNomadWisdom.com.

Muscle is the magic ingredient that has been missing from the recipe all along—the "yeast" designed to resurrect your muscles for the expansion of strength, growth, an entirely new way to live your life, and a whole new way to train your body. Soon, you will be stronger, fitter, and able to bound like a deer along your hiking path, climb a mountain, or just carry a bag of heavy groceries in from the car without any trouble at all. Yes, it *will* happen! Especially, when you begin training the right way.

Aerobic Exercise and the Mystical Calorie

There is nothing like watching that little number on the computer readout that stares back at you as it counts your calories on your recumbent bike, elliptical trainer, StairMaster, or treadmill. It slowly ticks upward as if to taunt your every move. Fifteen minutes on your recumbent bike, for example, might only yield you a burn of seventy-five calories—not even half that apple fritter you purchased this morning at Starbucks because you still seem to crave those sweets, and can't seem to find a way to make oatmeal in the morning, let alone eat it.

Calories are important, but what I want to do right now is put those little buggers in perspective. I want to put them where they belong. Help me gather them up, put them in a little fire pit and let's start burning them off one by one, even while we're sleeping next to that fire because that's what building muscle in your body will do. It will turn you into a living, breathing furnace—a metabolic machine able to burn fat, and leap tall buildings in a single bound. It is my hope that in the context of reading this book, you will finally understand why it's so important and how you can go about making it happen in a simple, straight-forward fashion.

The topic of strength training is covered in almost every book on fitness, every magazine article, every fitness segment on television, and every time your turn around, someone else has the "secret formula." Once again, the truth is there is no secret formula. The secret is in getting the work done and working the body scientifically, not for twelve weeks or eight weeks or in eight minutes a day, but for the rest of your life. And in every one of the years in the rest of your life, you are going to spend some serious time building strength and stimulating growth in your muscles as the foundation. If you're doing that, you almost can't go wrong with whatever else you're doing in between, as long as you're doing something. And something is strength training at least twice per week, and aerobic exercise three to six days a week.

In spite of the plethora of information on the subject of strength and muscle, I think its importance is still often missed. Like the outline of a beautiful human body behind sheer curtains—you can see the image, relish in its beauty, fantasize about what it would be like to be there next to it, yet you can't see the clear, focused picture. You can't touch it, feel it, or see the well-defined cuts of the shape. It's only a softened image, still unfocused—the most beautiful thing you've ever seen, and yet elusive. Everyone is talking about it and no one is willing to knock on the door. So let's knock, because I know we'll be invited in. We belong there.

Inside, on the other side of the curtains you discover a beautiful arrangement of the human body at work. A body at work and in motion moving heavy objects with grace and confidence. Like a factory at work all day long, the muscles of the body can and will work for you constantly. Your muscles will contract and relax, stretch and elongate—but only if you ask them to. Asking and acting is all you have to do. Just like knocking on that door. That beautiful image has been waiting inside for you, ready to share its essence, and longing to help you experience what life can really be like on the other side of those curtains.

Now, don't get too distracted. That beautiful being has work to do and so do you. And here's why.

The average 180-pound person will burn roughly three hundred calories per hour while walking, 284 if walking a twenty-minute mile, and 350 per hour if walking a fifteen-minute mile. That's pretty good, but again, there's more to the story.

While performing a good, well balanced, and significant strength training routine, this same person will burn up to 590 calories per hour. This also does not include what that same person burns in the recovery period. Most people are surprised to learn that you often burn more calories during the recovery phase of your strength workouts than you do while you're working. This is that controversial "after-burn" I referred to earlier in this book, and this is just one more of the secrets that have been held from you behind those curtains.

So, imagine this:

Taking a thirty to sixty-minute walk will help you burn 200 to 300 calories. Not bad, but it gets a lot better when you add some strength training.

Perform a circuit strength-training routine for thirty to sixty minutes and you will burn an additional 300 to 600 calories. Directly as a result of that strength training, you burn a few hundred more calories in your recovery later that evening while taking a nice hot bath and having a cup of Moroccan pomegranate red tea (let's say 300 more calories).

If you include the walk and the strength-training exercise together, that's anywhere from 800 to 1,200 calories for that one day of exercise. Not bad, and a heck of a lot better than the 75 to 150 you burned in 15 to 30 minutes on that recumbent bike, where every second felt like the ticking of a clock in your bedroom at night when you can't sleep, and where you are engaged in what is known as "non-weight-bearing exercise" because the bike is holding you up and, hence, you are not working against gravity, which would be so much better for your muscles and bones.

Even better, is that research shows that when you can generate at least a 1,500 calorie burn each week, that regardless of your nutrition, this amount of calorie burn is associated with weight loss. Here, in this example, you've just about done that in one day, and in large part as a result of adding the strength training exercise.

Even if you only did this twice per week, and then walked two to three more times, you would be on your way to crossing an important threshold as the curtains open and the beautiful image appears.

More importantly, you would now be building muscle—your most precious life asset. No, you can't wear it like a piece of jewelry, or sell it to the highest bidder for a profit. You can only bathe in its glow as it cranks up your metabolism one muscle myofilament at a time. Breeding each time you train, creating energy and vitality behind that curtain, and making you feel like one of the most powerful human beings on Earth, because now, you will be.

**Note: I realize at this point, you might be looking for the actual "formula" for this muscle-building work. I didn't leave it out completely. I wanted to do the subject true justice. So what I did instead is produce the formulas for you on that website I keep mentioning at www.FitnessNomadWisdom.com. Why? Because the most vital message in this book is the one about the importance of building muscle and what a difference-maker it is. Additionally, I find it almost useless when authors lay out training formulas in books, expecting you to take the text they've shared and put it to work for you. That just isn't going to work. It's too complicated and hard to follow in text form.

What I've created instead, on the website mentioned above, is a true Nomad Resource Center to help you tackle the work at hand. In addition, whether you hire me or some other fitness professional, I believe that in order to do this right and be successful, most people can't do it on their own.

So, I highly encourage you to take advantage of this resource, and start consuming everything I have put together for you there. I think you'll find that what I've put together is some of the most honest, straightforward, and useful content around. And of course, if you live locally in Madison, Wisconsin, or one of the surrounding areas, I would love to have you in my Nomad Kickstart Program. More information about that program can be found at: www.NomadKickstart.com.

The Top 5 Ways Strong Women and Men Make and Keep Strong Bones

In the early days of our space program, astronauts would return from space so weak that they couldn't walk. Often, they would need to be carried out of their flight capsules. Tests showed that they were losing significant amounts of bone and muscle mass while floating around Earth in space. These strong and vigorous men were losing 1 percent of their bone mass in only one week's time!

Your bones need gravity to survive and to thrive. Bones need regular exercise in the form of strength training. Inactivity and lack of exercise dissolves your bone mass. Does that sound appealing—your bones melting away like an Alka-Seltzer tablet in a glass of water? I wouldn't think so. The problem is that just like many other health problems such as high blood pressure, bone loss and osteoporosis are silent cripplers. They work underneath your radar, with jackhammers and backhoes while you sit, while you sleep, and definitely while you slip deeper and deeper into that couch and that lifetime full of so much inactivity.

Starting at the age of about thirty-five, you will begin losing about 1 percent of your bone mass each year. For women, during the year or two prior to menopause and for the first five years following this significant life change, women's estrogen levels drop and they experience an even more dramatic change in their bones. Void of the estrogen to contain them, the bone-dissolving osteoclasts increase their activity by about 20 percent. The osteoblasts that are responsible for laying down more bone don't increase to match this activity and the result is an increased net loss of bone. **Women can lose as much as 3 to 5 percent of their bone during this transformative time**, which is why this is such a critical time period for preventive measures. And bone loss continues at a rate of 1 to 2 percent from the post-menopause time period to the age of seventy.

By **age seventy, a woman may only have 60 to 70 percent of her bone mass left** and she becomes fragile and lives in a very dangerous state. Remember the story of my mother-in-law and her boot? By age eighty-five or ninety, a woman might only possess half of the bone mass she had at her peak! Not a great foundation for keeping up with the grandkids or staying out of the nursing home.

The Good News

The good news is that if you take action, you can prevent much of this loss. And even if you're already living with some degree of osteoporosis and bone loss, at least some of those changes can be reversed. Strength training twice a week, for example, dramatically cuts the risk of fractures in postmenopausal women. Numerous studies have confirmed that well designed strength training programs build bone.

Muscles are attached to your bones with tendons. As your muscles work and contract, those tendons tug on your bones and stimulate growth. The stronger your muscles, the greater force created when they tug, and the more bone you build. This is another very important reason that at least four times a year, you spend time building strength and growth in your muscles.

5 Things You Can Do to Maintain Strong Bones for Life

Do bone-building strength training at least twice, if not three times per week. As described in the paragraph above, a well-designed strength training program stimulates bone growth. This program should include specific exercises for the hips, spine, and arms because these areas are more prone to fractures. For now, and until you can have someone design a program for you, vertical jumping just two minutes per day as been shown in the research to have a positive effect on building and maintaining your bones. In addition, researchers have also found that high-impact activities like tennis, volleyball, basketball, jumping rope, and jumping jacks can also help to improve bone much more quickly. When you perform these exercises, your bones are subjected to forces that are three to six times greater than your body weight.

Your strength-training program also needs to be of an adequate intensity level to build bone mass. Generally speaking, you should do one exercise for each major muscle group of the body and perform two to three sets of eight to twelve repetitions of each exercise. And you should feel like you really couldn't do more than twelve repetitions. Keep in mind that you may need to work into a program like this slowly, and that, if you're are just starting out, higher repetition ranges (fifteen to twenty reps for example) for about a four-week time period, is paramount for building an adequate foundation from which you can push harder. The best thing to do is to hire a professional fitness trainer to help at least get you started. There is NO substitute for this.

Dispel the myth that might exist in your mind that walking, swimming, and biking are the best exercises for preventing and treating osteoporosis. It is true that women with a life-long habit of walking have a 30 percent lower fracture rate than women who don't. And walking is great exercise, but it is not nearly enough to stimulate significant bone growth. Even a year-long walking program has been shown to have little effect on your bones.

Swimming and biking are even less effective than walking because they are non-weight-bearing activities. The water and the bike are holding your body weight. And having to fight with gravity is the key to your bone growth. Remember the astronauts?

Good Nutrition. You may already have a good nutrition program, but often it might need major adjustments for optimal bone benefits. Calcium usually gets all the attention, but vitamin D is potentially more vital than calcium. Its presence is essential for optimal absorption of calcium. And, of course, plenty of fruits and vegetables, vitamin C, magnesium, and potassium, and soy protein is also showing promise.

Getting enough protein and eating a well-balanced diet is also essential to stimulating the strength and growth in your muscles that, in turn, affects the health of your bones. You must eat to grow and thrive. And that eating must be balanced and full of fresh whole foods, and the essential vitamins and minerals important for bone and muscle growth.

Stop Looking at Osteoporosis as an Old Lady's Disease. Many younger women ignore recommendations for building and maintaining bone because they think of the problem as one that only affects women and men who are much older. The truth is that the process of bone dissolution can begin very early in life. As stated earlier, once you hit the age of thirty-five, look out! You are likely not to feel the effects until later in life, but your bones are melting while you're not looking. So get to work!

Never Give up or Give In. Most people believe that once the process of bone loss has occurred and someone has been diagnosed with osteoporosis, there is nothing they can do about it. Quite the contrary. You're not going to recover *all* of the bone you've lost, but the latest treatments can actually restore bone. And even small gains in bone density can make a meaningful difference in preventing fractures.

In addition, there is a growing body of research that demonstrates the ability of women and men in their sixties, seventies, and eighties who are still able to grow bone when they begin a well-designed strength and conditioning program. The body is always willing to get stronger—you simply have to ask it to work for you.

More Muscle Equals More Metabolic Activity

More Strength, and More Bone:
The Key Ingredients for a Strong & Productive Life

You should now understand that muscle is significantly more active metabolically than fat tissue, and takes up much less space in the body. One pound of muscle is about the size of a baseball and will burn thirty-five to fifty calories per day, which is the equivalent of more than five pounds of body fat per year.

This might not sound like a lot to you. In fact, I'm almost sure it doesn't because these are the kinds of conversations I have with clients all day long. The drive for the quick and easy solution to your problems is tempting, seductive, and enticing, and at the same time impossible if you're really doing it right. Building muscle takes a transformation of your physiology and it takes time. It also takes very good nutrition habits, because if you're not feeding your body properly in the recovery process from your strength workouts, you're severing the body's ability to recover, get stronger, and grow.

So, let's go back to that five pounds a year and your commitment to the journey. Regular exercise is a lifetime sport. You don't get to give it up, take a break, or even stop for a little while. The work is on-going and an essential part of life, like eating. You won't live very long if you don't eat. If you don't build muscle, you still might live long, but it is likely to feel like twice as long. You'll be miserable during the last one third of your existence, and your body will not continue to allow you to do the things you really want to do, like staying lean and self-reliant.

That said, I think the five pounds per year starts to make a little more sense. If you're in this for the long run, for every pound of muscle you build, you'll burn an extra five pounds of fat per year, every year until you're lean again. Assuming you don't quit, give up, or shy away from the kind of serious strength and growth-building exercises that I'm recommending in this book.

So, let's just say, for instance, that you have thirty-five pounds to lose and that you are serious about making it happen. Let's also say that you're adding a pound of muscle about twice per year—two pounds per year (a conservative and realistic estimate). In about three and a half years, you'll have the extra muscle you need to keep those thirty-five pounds away for good. Yes, I can hear you from here. "Three and a half years to lose thirty-five pounds? That's ridiculous!" Well, actually it is, because if you're serious about what you're doing, it will happen a lot faster than that, especially if you're focused on building strength and growth in your muscles, eating strategically, and doing your cardiovascular exercise. But I wanted to make a point, and my experience during the last seven years in particular has shown me that most people just aren't able to take enough of the serious kind of action necessary to generate faster results. Weight loss is a big job, good habits take time to form, and most people struggle in the first 6 months to a year of their work because of that. If they stick with it, they learn how to build a healthier lifestyle. If they get impatient, they quit and NEVER gain success, hence the articles you find about how weight loss is hard, or impossible, and so often reversed if it even happens in the first place. Remember, this is for the rest of your life.

My point is that if you put this in its proper perspective, and think about how many years it took you to park those thirty-five pounds of fat securely into your belly, and you think about the .3 to .5 percent of muscle loss you've had each year since you turned thirty-five, and you're fifty years old today, three and a half years is nothing! Most people, by the time they arrive in that little red chair in my office, have been laying down the groundwork for their fat farm for ten, fifteen, or twenty years. That's a dramatic change in the physiology of the body, and being able to reverse it in just three years is pretty good.

Can you make it happen faster? Absolutely, yes. I've seen it happen; and if you're interested, you can watch Sara's video on the success stories page at www.TheFitnessNomad.com for a great example of what happens when you truly apply yourself. But it's a rarity, especially if you want to keep that weight off for good. Still, it's possible, and Sara is an awesome example! I highly encourage you to watch her story; it's incredibly informative and inspiring.

We're all now familiar with the idea that people lose weight and gain it back within a year or two. You've likely seen this happen with someone you know or your own efforts. If you are able to take quick and efficient action, and you are able to make your thirty-five pounds of fat disappear more quickly, then please make sure you're doing it right. Doing it right means building strength, building muscles, and building bones, and not relying exclusively on your scale for tracking results. If your weight on the scale is dropping and is not accompanied by a proportionate drop in your body fat, then you are muscle wasting and that is a recipe for long-term struggle with your weight.

Your muscles are your assets and once you build them and commit to maintaining them, they are working for you 24/7. And I'll repeat it because it's so important. When I say "doing it right and not relying on the scale," what I mean is that when you do this weight loss thing wrong, your scale is more than willing to lie to you. Weight loss on the scale is not enough. Your weight loss *must* be accompanied by a concurrent reduction in your body fat percentage. If the two are not coming down together at the right relative rates, you're muscle wasting. That's an even more dangerous situation than all that fat hanging around in your belly. It sets you up for more failure in the long run. More failure means more fat and a situation where you reach a point of no return. I covered this in more detail in the Problem Section of this book, under the chapter titled, "Your Scale is Lying to You." There are also a number of videos on my YouTube channel that address this subject in particular (www.YouTube.com/fitnessnomad).

So, instead of beginning this journey from the land of denial and misinformation, and with an unrealistic viewpoint of what your body is actually capable of, and of what creates lasting change, let's begin from the point of acceptance, forgiveness, and surrender.

It's okay that you let it slide for so long. You need to forgive yourself for that one. But it's not okay to continue sliding, because the mud pit at the bottom is thick, dirty, ugly, and very difficult to climb out of. That's why you've reached this point in the book and that's why you've decided to do something about it. The important part is that you have decided to make this a life commitment—a commitment to yourself, your humanity, and the legend of strength that we are all responsible for maintaining.

No longer will the world be so full of people who hide in denial and allow themselves to accept the false belief that being overweight, unfit, weak, and fat is a by-product of the aging process. No longer will you hide from the serious work waiting for you in the gym, behind those curtains, and in a place that builds so much more than strength and muscle. From now on, you are taking full responsibility for this legend and you will do your part to help it unfold in a much more inspiring way.

You now know that choosing this path takes commitment, hard work, dedication, and discipline. When you hit roadblocks and smash into barriers, you will also commit to them as part of the journey and your growth as a human being—a being with an unrelenting and deep-rooted desire to be stronger, fitter, and more muscular.

Muscle and Its Affect on Your Bones

More muscle equals more bone. It really is that simple. Bones grow when muscles tug on them during exercise. The bigger and stronger your muscles are, the more you stimulate bone growth. Once again, more bone tissue also means more work for the body physiologically. It also means that in addition to all of your muscle mass, you also now have even stronger bones holding them up. All of which makes you stronger, more powerful, and increasingly more able to progress your fitness program.

Remember that concept of Progressive Overload I introduced in the chapter on strength? Progressive Overload is the key to building strength and muscle in the body. Progressive Overload is placing increasingly more difficult stress on the body on a regular basis, so the body has to continue to adapt and overcome and ultimately become stronger and more fit. The stronger your foundation becomes, the better you are able to do this.

The bottom line here is that you're either growing or decaying and dying like a wilting flower in the summer sun. All you really need is a little water on a regular basis so that you can solidify your roots and exist like the bean stalk instead of the wilting flower.

Building Muscle is a Lifelong Process

As I mentioned earlier in this chapter and throughout this book, you need to be committed for the long run and committed to building strength and growth in your muscles at least four times a year. The journey never ends, it only changes, adapts, and meanders through your lifetime. Here are a couple of examples. The second one is quite personal.

This morning I raced home from my usual Wednesday morning networking meeting. I had taken some extra time to connect with some of the other folks, which cramped my time a bit. But that was okay because part of what I had the chance to do was let someone tell me how much I've inspired him since joining the group six months ago. He is not a client, but has watched me jumping around in front of the group every week, felt my presence in the room, and let me point him down the path of strength and fitness. He is now swimming regularly every morning at 5:30 and his knees don't ache as they did a month ago. His pants fit a little better and his energy level has improved. For him, this is excellent progress and a great start. It was great to hear his story. It was a good example of the meandering and at the very least, a start.

More personally, on that same day, I was racing home to pick up my laptop and bag, along with some food, so that I could get to the studio early enough to work out. I had gained great momentum with my own fitness program, and at the time a better looking body at the pool was my own vain external motivation. I was not going to miss an opportunity to lift some heavy weight that day. I was looking forward to the chance to challenge a body that was feeling increasingly strong, fit, and inspired. I always accomplish more in the gym on days like that. I don't always feel that way—sometimes, it's exactly the opposite—but I always keep going.

The way I felt that day didn't happen overnight. The process had been unfolding over many years, and is the culmination of a lifetime commitment to exercise that is undying. I have heard strength defined as the ability to confront pain and stick with it. If you've experienced pain yourself, you know exactly what I'm talking about. And if you're human, there's almost no way you haven't experienced both physical and emotional pain. Often, it's the emotional pain that builds the true and lasting inner strength that manifests in the physical realm; but only if you'll allow it to help you do so.

Strength is built in many ways. What we build in strength physically dances graciously with the strength we have and build emotionally. They take turns leading. Neither is in control all of the time. This is because one feeds the other, much like a baby who feeds its mother with unconditional love and trust, while the mother provides food, shelter, and an extension of what fed that baby in the womb.

Strength cannot be borrowed or bought or even stolen, and your search for it and work for it are never done. It is in this unending journey that more of it is discovered and with each new dig, each new plateau overcome, each new personal best achieved, and each new muscle identified in the mirror, both your physical and emotional strength increase. Each increase makes you a more and more powerful human being.

On this journey, you are always growing, expanding, contracting, and exploring new territory in your mind, your muscles, your body, and beyond. And as long as you stay grounded most of the time in the work that your body is capable of today, you chart the territory you need to chart each day, recover, grow, and expand. You grow like a flower in unexpected and beautiful ways. While you sometimes follow the path of least resistance, the time you spend in the work of building your body and strengthening your mind takes you down the path of most resistance. It is along this path that I believe we find ourselves, grow, and make our own personal contribution to the legend of humankind.

Remember . . .

Your Strength Endures as Legend—
You Must Fight!

"If you've read this entire book cover to cover, you will see that this small section at the end is a repeat of an earlier section. I've included it here again both because it's my favorite passage of the book, and possibly the most important. It is also the part of this book I'm most hopeful about. It is a passage I hope will inspire you and encourage you to begin your own journey as part of this legend, and then share it with me, so that together we can inspire others. I, of course, am attached to this passage because it is mine, and I wrote it straight from my heart. As a result, I also chose to finish this book—my first book—with its words. I hope you enjoy it as much as I do . . . "—John

Building strength and stimulating growth in your muscles is on-going, never-ending—a timeless project that builds the legend of humankind.

Sound daunting? Good, that means you're growing—not just growing muscle, but growing as a human being.

One day I was working out in my fitness studio. Working on this thing called muscles—my assets. The experience was thrilling. Yes, thrilling. The feeling of moving heavy iron and weight through the atmosphere, around in space, up and down, and through my body is cleansing, like taking a hot bath from the inside out.

At one point, I asked one of the trainers who worked for me at the time, Kirk, for a spot on the bench press and I realized something very important—something I know instinctively, yet it still needed to be reinforced. No matter how hard you've worked, or how tired your body might feel, there is always more work and more growth possible. All you have to do is ask.

"How many are you doing?" Kirk asked.

"Not more than five." I replied. I then proceeded to lift the bar from the rack, my feet in the air, my core and trunk engaged like a lion on the hunt, and began moving the weight up and down.

"Good!" Kirk encouraged at just the right time. "Strong, breathe. Inhale" (as the bar moved down), "breathe" (as I pushed the bar up).

When I reached the down-stroke of rep number five I was on my way to a job well done.

"Okay, keep going," Kirk encouraged.

And I did, only because he asked me to and I agreed in an instant that more was possible. The set ended with eight repetitions and the last two were like a fog rolling into the San Francisco Bay, mysterious and sudden and numbing in a good way—a soft, cool blanket that is refreshing in its surprise.

Kirk wanted me to do nine, but I was already finished in my mind. As I reflected on the experience, I decided that if I had stayed strong in my head, one more (possibly with a little help from Kirk) would have been possible. I say "strong in my mind" because that strength reaches out to the rest of the body like an old friend after a year of absence.

I've heard another say that strength can endure like a legend, even beyond our lifetime. I think this is true because there's something that happens when you go into that fog of the work—that misty place where almost anything is possible, like the growth of the legendary bean stalk into the clouds. It's that place where time stands still and once and for all your body takes on its own agenda—an agenda that exists beyond conscious thought, somewhere deep in the DNA where your physiology cries out for more because that's what it is built for.

You can't buy or borrow it. You can only cultivate your body's innate willingness to build it, like the mastermind behind the skyscraper that almost seems to erect itself. The vision of what your body needs and craves is always present. When we ground ourselves in the kiva, hold heavy things until our muscles burn in delight, we tap into that vision that is lying dormant in our DNA, hiding from us—the vision our Creator had for us all along to be strong, pursue our evolution like dynamos, and build a better and stronger body as a foundation.

To build this kind of strength, you need patience, understanding, and self-love. You can't let your head and the thoughts that build storms there, hinder your progress, and infect your DNA with the virus of weakness that only exists when you are not grounded enough to feel the truth digging deep into the earth from your feet. Building strength and muscle does not come quickly and your work is never done because the work of your evolution is never done.

Overnight strength is mirage, a trick of the body's neurological system, a quick adaptation designed to allow you to accomplish more—if you're willing to perform the work and dig the trenches. Eighty percent of your strength gains at any one given time are primarily a result of the increased efficiency of your neurological system. It is a more efficient recruitment of motor units that innervate your muscles and ask them to contract. This is an exquisite process and a symbol of the universal plan for all of us to evolve, grow, and be strong. This is the human body in the heat of the work it was designed to do all along. We have simply lost touch with this truth in our cubicles and sedentary lives along the way, as we attempt to find solace in Dilbert, when instead we should have been looking for it in that gym downstairs—the one the wellness committee built for us a year ago and that no one is using.

This adaptation of the nervous system is important because it helps us build the foundation we need to keep going, keep working, and ultimately keep growing muscle. Yet, it will only happen if we are working hard enough and often enough to feed the roots.

Staying in those high repetition ranges where the weight is light and the fog is thin—if present at all—is nice. What we really need to do is conquer the fear that comes with the thicker fog—the one that only allows us to see a few feet ahead of us. This is a fog that forces us to trust the work and ourselves and that allows us to believe that lifting more weight is not only possible, but thrilling. It is the foghorn under your feet on the Golden Gate Bridge.

Lifting more weight is also essential to stimulate muscle growth. If 80 percent of your gains in muscle strength can be attributed to motor learning, this means that 80 percent of your strength gains are due primarily to your nervous system's ability to recruit muscle fibers that were not previously being used, and learning to use those fibers in more efficient ways.

This is good news for all aspects of your training and fitness, but it is also the same reason that most people often hit those dreaded plateaus where they experience diminishing returns for the time they spend at the gym. This is especially true for women who tend to lift in higher repetition ranges and with lighter weights. Muscle gets stronger (to a point), especially early in a training program. If a new and more significant stimulus is not applied, however, it begins to lie dormant, like a hidden treasure at the bottom of the sea. Only a brave and well-planned exploration can dig it up.

This exploration is your willingness to start training your muscles in a new and much more challenging way, at least four times a year. Unless you do, you will continue to experience less and less return on your investment of time, and soon will find yourself wondering why you decided to do this work in the first place.

Your exploration will take you on a search for the treasure that is waiting for you deep in the core of every one of your muscles. Those cells and your DNA have been waiting for you to begin digging—to begin the journey of unlocking the codes that will stimulate your muscles to grow. Your muscles will grow like a tulip in early spring, moving first a little slow as the ground continues to warm, poking its head cautiously above the earth. And then, as the sun shines and it is fed, it too taps into the roots of its DNA and the resulting photosynthesis allows it to grow toward the sky, bloom, and provide leadership for the rest of spring.

Your muscles hold those same codes, those same memories from other lifetimes where gladiators tapped in to the source and used it to fight until their death. Like it or not, you too are fighting until your death in a different way. Like it or not, your muscles and bones will either grow or die and once you hit the age of thirty to forty, they begin that process of death and wearing out. But they won't if you fight like the warrior in the coliseum—not if you fight.

You must first fight to unlock the potential of your muscles. You must cut through the fog and break down your barriers, like that warrior entering the stadium. Break yourself free from the shackles that have been tied to your ankles by a culture's move away from the physical activity and work that our DNA demands. Then, you must fight every day for the work your muscles desire in the gym—the work that stimulates their growth, your growth, and your strength and the strength of the world as legend.

The Fitness Nomad Wisdom Center

Okay, you've finished the book. Way to go! I hope you enjoyed reading it as much as I enjoyed writing it.

I referred often to The Fitness Nomad Wisdom Center online at www.FitnessNomadWisdom.com because once I got going on this book, I quickly realized that creating this resource center was an important part of this work—work I've done for you and all those wanting to improve their lives.

There is a ton of great stuff there, and if you're one of the first to invest in the book, you'll get immediate access to the wisdom center for FREE.

All you have to do is visit www.FitnessNomadWisdom.com and click the link you see in the right hand column of the page that reads,

"Already Purchased The Book? Click Here"

That link will take you to a short form where you can enter the following code and be granted immediate access:

"be a fitness nomad"

There is a ton of great stuff already there, and I will continue to add to it throughout the rest of the year and with each new Fitness Nomad Book of Wisdom.

I hope to see you there soon . . . —John